D0175774

The Intrinsic Exerciser

The
Intrinsic
Exerciser

Discovering
the
Joy of Exercise

Jay Kimiecik

Houghton Mifflin Company
Boston · New York   2002

Copyright © 2002 by Jay Kimiecik
All rights reserved

For information about permission to reproduce selections
from this book, write to Permissions, Houghton Mifflin Company,
215 Park Avenue South, New York, New York 10003.

Visit our Web site: www.houghtonmifflinbooks.com.

Library of Congress Cataloging-in-Publication Data
Kimiecik, Jay
The Intrinsic Exerciser : Discovering the Joy of
Exercise / Jay Kimiecik.
p.   cm.
Includes bibliographical references and index.
ISBN 0-618-12490-X
1. Physical fitness — Psychological aspects.
2. Exercise — Psychological aspects. 3. Health
psychology. I. Title.
RA781.K536 2002
613.7—dc21   2001051887

Printed in the United States of America

Book design by Robert Overholtzer

QUM 10 9 8 7 6 5 4 3 2 1

Portions of this book were adapted from material that originally
appeared in a series of articles in *IDEA Health and Fitness Source*,
Psychology Today, a chapter on flow written with Susan Jackson
in *Advances in Sport Psychology*, ed. Thelma S. Horn (2nd ed.),
and the YMCA of the USA's *YPersonal Fitness Program:
12 Weeks to a Better You Program Manual*.

For my wife, Kim

my one and only boilermaker

Acknowledgments

This book is the result of living the life of an intrinsic athlete, exerciser, worker, husband, and parent for many years. I have many people to thank for that.

From the academic side of things, I've been fortunate to have many mentors who were willing to listen to my intrinsic way of looking at the world — Maria Allison, Joan Duda, Glyn Roberts, Ed McAuley, and Rainer Martens, to name just a few. I want to thank them for giving me an opportunity to explore ideas in my own way. I am forever grateful. Special thanks to my department chair at Miami University, Robin Vealey, who understood my need for isolation and made sure I had an office to write this book during renovation chaos. Thanks also to Thelma Horn, who has been a wonderful research collaborator.

As I have progressed in my career, many people in the real world have helped me spread my wings outside the Ivory Tower of academia. Mike Spezzano of the YMCA of

Acknowledgments

the USA gave me a chance to contribute to the development and writing of the *YPersonal Fitness Program*. Thanks to Dick Webster and Jennifer Bolger, who adapted my behavior change ideas into a breakthrough exercise behavior change program. And special thanks to Carrie Phelps and Joann Donnelly, who have been a source of inspiration with their commitment to health and fitness in their work with the YMCA.

And to all my FitLinxx, Inc., friends — Keith Camhi, Andy Greenberg, Anita Anderson, and many others — thank you for giving me the chance to express my views and opinions on exercise at many seminars around the country. Those experiences have helped me live my dream and fine-tune the Intrinsic Exerciser approach to exercise behavior change. Please continue the fitness revolution.

I wouldn't have learned as much about motivation and behavior change without some great graduate students at Miami University: Laura Hoag, Moe Swift, Jill Dempsey, Dawn Anderson Butcher, Amy Harris, Stacy Wegley, Bryan Blissmer, Jen Wren, April White, and Luann Reddecliff. And thanks to all of the awesome undergraduate students at Miami, especially Shannon Prince, who someday will be a great something. And I have already learned tons from the next generation of Intrinsic Exercisers: Merrin Jump and Joyce Englander.

I received much professional help in writing this book. I want to thank Diane Lofshult, editor of *IDEA Health and Fitness Source*, who was the first one to give me the opportunity to publish my Intrinsic Exerciser ideas in a

Acknowledgments

somewhat practical format. Thanks also to Camille Chatterjee, formerly of *Psychology Today*, who was the second. With their assistance, I was able to see the possibilities for the Intrinsic Exerciser. Thanks to all of the folks at Houghton Mifflin Company who from the beginning believed in me and the book. Special thanks to Susan Canavan, Bridget Marmion, and Lori Glazer for guiding me through the publishing process. I greatly appreciate their commitment to making this book as good as it gets. Special, special thanks to Laura van Dam, my editor, who always encouraged me and whose insight into the practical aspects of exercise made the final product far better than I ever imagined.

A special thank-you to John Hingsbergen at Miami University National Public Radio WMUB for giving me a chance to break into radio with the *FitTalk* show and *The Fitness Minute*. I have learned a great deal about exercise and motivation and met some great people through hosting the show.

Over the years, some close friends pulled me through so that I could get to the point of writing a book. Gene Babon believed in me when most others didn't; Gary Stein helped me keep things in perspective; Sue Jackson showed me what commitment to work is all about; and Doug Newburg has helped me revisit, and then live, the real Dream that is inside me. I also want to thank all of the people I have met through the Resonance Group. I have been touched by all of you. Long live resonance!

A special thank-you to all of the folks who participated in our Intrinsic Exerciser e-mail group. The stories they

Acknowledgments

were willing to share about exercise and their lives were poignant, thought-provoking, and brought the Intrinsic Exerciser to life for me. I look forward to learning more from all of them. I want to especially thank the people whose stories ended up in this book: Anita Anderson, Kristi Nadler, Keely K., Frank Roberts, and Rita Callahan. Thank you all for your honesty, authenticity, and willingness to share, and to inspire others.

Besides my family, the one person who is most responsible for getting this book into print is my agent, Jenny Bent. It was her belief, support, and tenacity that convinced the folks at Houghton Mifflin of the merits of the Intrinsic Exerciser concept. Without Jenny, I'd still be writing the proposal or getting rejection letters. Thanks, Jenny.

Thanks to my family: Mom, Dad, Greg, Sandy, and Kathy. I am who I am because of the life I led before I left for the great unknown more than 20 years ago. You all somehow instilled in me a joy and passion for life and movement that I can't explain but am forever thankful for. Dad, thanks for playing sports with me all those years, and, Mom, thanks for showing me what it means to be a hero. Greg, you gave me the heart to go one-on-one with anyone. Sandy, your willingness to express your views and opinions keeps my mind sharp. And, Kathy, you've helped me become more convinced that the Dream is inside everyone. And thanks, Sandy, for the writing house, and thanks, Mom and Dad, for letting me write portions of this book in the very room in which I grew up. Special thanks to Grandma Kimiecik, who gave me the gift of

Acknowledgments

storytelling. And I must thank Chris Colyer, whose commitment to our children is a miracle.

To my wife, Kim, and our two children, Carly and Colin, thank you for allowing me to hold on to my intrinsic self in all areas of my life. Kim, your commitment to our life together — and keeping the fun — has fueled my fire to keep going at times when I needed it the most. You have helped me hold on to my dream and develop new ones. Without you I would be sucked up by extrinsicness and meaninglessness. And thank you for saving our children for me. Carly and Colin, your enthusiasm for learning, exploring, and moving provided the continual evidence and support that I was onto something. And thank you for interrupting my writing all of those times. How did you know I needed a play break? I look forward to many more intrinsic fun times with you and your mother. Play on so we can all turn into rainbows!

Contents

Contents

Foreword

Books about what's good for us tend to be mechanical and boring. Beside, most of them are wrong. Oh, their intentions are usually excellent and their facts often correct, but they overlook the essential point. Whether the book tries to get you to eat a healthier diet, exercise more, or get along with your spouse and children, it doesn't acknowledge that people won't switch to a healthier behavior just because it's good for them — unless the decision to do so fits their life goals, and provides enjoyment.

The Intrinsic Exerciser does not make this mistake. The book is theoretically sound — which academicians like me appreciate — but more important, it is full of common sense, and it's fun to read. The four steps it presents — physical activity, a natural expression of our evolutionary past, should become part of our self-image; we should use our bodies as a tool for exercising mastery; we should enjoy this mastery in the moment, not for external reasons like health or reducing weight; and finally, it should become an integral part of our daily life so it generates "Inergy" — are both feasible and necessary to sustain a continuing physical regimen. Health and fitness will follow, but they are not what sustains the exercise of the body.

This is an honest book. It doesn't promise instant results, it does not suggest that living a healthy life in the 21st century is easy. It may be difficult, but it need not be a chore. In fact, once you understand how using the body's potential can become part of your mental and spiritual life, physical exercise can become a constant source of some of your most exhilarating and memorable moments. One would hope that most readers will take the time to reflect on what this book is saying and make it part of their daily routines. But even if one chooses not to apply its advice, it will provide useful understanding into our physical nature, and an enjoyable read.

Mihaly Csikszentmihalyi
Hamilton, Montana, 2001

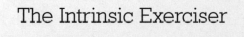

The Intrinsic Exerciser

Introduction

You picked this book, so you must have some interest in exercise. Maybe you have even tried to exercise regularly in the past. Perhaps you thought exercise could help you lose some weight, but even that desire wasn't strong enough for you to stay with it. You may have a piece of exercise equipment somewhere in your house that is serving as a form of interior design. You may have watched exercise infomercials. You may have bought the tapes. You may have read the best-selling health and fitness books, which assume that losing weight and reducing your risk of disease are the main reasons you should exercise. I have nothing against the authors, but they are wrong, wrong in the sense that people don't exercise for those reasons. These books are packed with information that doesn't motivate or inspire you to truly change, to transform yourself into a regular exerciser. Reading these books, you tell yourself that this is it, now is the time I will start and maintain an exercise program. But a few months later, even the best intentions have turned into guilt, frustration, and minimal movement. Like the deer in the headlights, your body remains motionless. You may feel better to know that you are not alone: studies show that millions of people have had similar experiences.

The answer to how to become a regular exerciser is simple but one that most people haven't heard or thought much about. *To become a regular exerciser over a long period of time, you must learn to love moving your body.* That's it! And to enjoy moving your body you must develop what I call the *intrinsic mindset* for changing behavior. Frankly, helping people find the joy or passion in movement is what's missing from most of the programs and books you may have tried. Intrinsic motivation — performing a task primarily for its own sake — is the most powerful way to change behavior, yet few health and fitness programs or infomercials ever tell you about it.

I'm here to tell you that it's possible and absolutely necessary over the long haul for you to love your exercise. Don't believe 'em when "the experts" tell you to exercise even if you don't like it because it's "good for you." You *don't* become a regular exerciser by telling yourself it will help you lose weight or reduce your risk of disease. You can only drag yourself to the gym for so long without enjoying it. Going on sheer willpower or guilt is not enough to make you change. Yet that is the message you typically hear from the health and fitness profession and the media. Instead, you become an exerciser by finding the joy and fun before, during, and after every exercise experience. People who have become regular exercisers know all about this intrinsic approach, and I'm sharing this best-kept secret with you here. It's a simple but different approach to exercise that is fun and effective.

You may be a little skeptical. But consider this: if all of the existing weight loss and exercise programs are so great, why do scientific data show an alarming rise in overweight individuals in this country over the past 20 years? Why are there millions of physically inactive people, as reported in *Physical Activity and Health: A Report of the Surgeon General*? More fitness information and exercise equipment are available now than ever before, but people's health habits are getting worse. Could it be that this information is so far removed from your inner experience with your own body that it is meaningless? When is the last time you were really aware of your body in motion? When is the last time you felt the joy of movement? This book helps you turn inward, to change your exercise behavior from the inside out and in the process become what I call an Intrinsic Exerciser.

I'll be honest with you. I don't have a personal weight loss success story to throw at you. I don't have a "program" in my back pocket to sell you. However, I have moved my body on a regular basis since I was old enough to crawl — going on about 43 years. And I've been lucky enough to devote the past 15 years to studying why people exercise and why they don't. I've learned a few things about myself and other regular exercisers during this journey that I believe can help you exercise because you want to.

If you are tired of yo-yo exercising — sporadic spurts of

movement mixed with long periods of inactivity — this book is for you. If you've joined all of the gyms listed in your Yellow Pages, this book can help. If you've made more attempts to exercise than the number of rock-hard abdominal machines on the market, it's probably time to take the inner path to regular exercise. But this book isn't just for the sporadic exerciser. If you are one of the few who already exercise on a regular basis, you can also benefit by learning more about how to enjoy exercise for its own sake. It will rekindle the fire and inspire you to continue. In essence, this book is for anyone who wants to become an Intrinsic Exerciser, the purest form of motivating yourself to exercise on a regular basis.

I start off by helping you understand the typical approach — Outside-In — that people use to exercise and why it's not very effective. Then I move to the Inside-Out approach, and I help you take the four inner steps to developing the mindset of an Intrinsic Exerciser. Finally, I explore how to apply your intrinsic mindset to overcome some of the barriers to exercise that you face every day.

A Short Note on What This Book Is Not

Before you read any further, I must warn you that this book is different from other books on exercise. Here are some of the things it *will not do:*

- It won't outline the relationships among exercise, fitness, weight, and disease reduction.

- It won't explain the physiological benefits of exercise.

- It won't explain how to develop cardiovascular endurance, muscular strength and endurance, and flexibility.

- It won't address eating behavior or weight loss, at least not directly.

- It won't explain how exercise can reduce the risk of cancer, prevent osteoporosis, or influence other chronic degenerative diseases.

- It won't advocate a "canned" or "cookie cutter" behavior change program of any kind.

There are many good sources of information on how to start an exercise program, guidelines for getting fit, the proper way to lose weight, and so on. But they haven't helped you change your behavior, have they? In fact, overemphasizing these aspects of exercise gets in the way of developing authentic motivation for change.

The main purpose of this book is to help you change your mindset about yourself and exercise so that you'll maximize the enjoyment of moving your body. The book helps you develop a set of inner skills that will radically change the way you think and feel about yourself and exercise. In this transformation, you will forge your own inner path to movement, which will stay with you for the rest of your life.

How to Use This Book

The book offers you the inner resources and tools to help you make a motivational or mindset shift in how you think about and experience exercise. You make that shift by working on the four steps to becoming an Intrinsic Exerciser: Vision, Mastery, Flow, and Inergy. The sequence of the chapters is based on my experience and understanding of how people have become Intrinsic Exercisers.

As you progress, try at least one practical strategy from each chapter. Don't just read the material and put the book away. Shifting your mindset from extrinsic to intrinsic will occur only if you work with the material and make connections to your own situation. Whether you have been physically active your whole life or thinking about it or somewhere in between, something is here for you.

Get Ready to Discover Your Intrinsic Exerciser

Within each of us is a mover, an exerciser. For some of us this inner mover is deeper inside than for others. But all of us can reach it — some will just have to peel off more layers. Our bodies were made to be physically active, to move for their own sake. You need only watch preschoolers at a playground for a short while to know this truth. If you ask these children why they move their bodies so passionately, they look at you as if you were from another planet, then run off to swing on the monkey bars for the umpteenth time. I bet you forgot that you and I were once those children. It's time to remember.

Part I

....

Moving from Outside-In to Inside-Out

1
....

Outside-In: The Extrinsic Approach to Exercise

> Those who cannot change their minds cannot change anything.
>
> — George Bernard Shaw

By now you've heard or read most of the reasons that you should be physically active. You know at some level that exercise is a great way to lose weight. Exercise can also help you live longer as well as reduce your risk of certain kinds of diseases, such as coronary artery disease, obesity, diabetes, and osteoporosis. The complete list of the benefits of exercise is longer than the ride lines at Disney World.

So why are so few people exercising? Well, most folks say they don't have enough time, don't know how, or that the effort is too much. In fact, most people just don't have the right mindset for exercising because they've been brainwashed by what I call the Outside-In approach to behavior change. For example, most of us focus on exercise as a way to look good, be fit, or lose weight — ideas that focus on the outcome of exercising. Therefore, they don't have a lot of motivational impact.

The Outside-In approach focuses on the logical and rational reasons that you should exercise. Outside-In emphasizes things outside yourself; the reasons and benefits of exercise come from external sources, which lead us away from the exercise experience itself. On the surface, the reasons are good. Who doesn't want to reduce the risk of coronary artery disease? Who doesn't want to live longer? Who doesn't want to lose some weight? Ironically, the onslaught of focusing on these external factors may even have the reverse effect on people: they make us less likely to become regular exercisers, which leads to more people being overweight and having a greater risk of suffering diseases.

If the Outside-In approach worked, 98 percent of the people who spend billions of dollars on weight loss products and programs wouldn't gain the weight back or add even more pounds within six months to a year. And the number of obese people in the United States wouldn't have risen from 12 percent in 1991 to 18 percent in 1998, resembling a communicable disease epidemic. The incidence of diabetes would not have increased by 6 percent in 1999, which led the director of the Centers for Disease Control, Jeffrey Koplan, to state, "This dramatic new evidence signals the unfolding of an epidemic in the United States." Approximately 300,000 Americans would not die prematurely each year due to physical inactivity and poor nutrition. The

Outside-In approach to lifestyle change is literally a dead-end street.

The effects of the Outside-In approach are summed up by a CDC epidemiologist, Ali Mokdad: "The message is out there: lose weight by increasing your physical activity and changing your diet. But nobody is doing it." That's because the message doesn't connect with your mind, heart, and soul. The Outside-In approach to behavior change has no staying power. You don't transform your thoughts and feelings to make exercise an enjoyable and uplifting experience.

Why Outside-In Rules

Almost without your knowing it, Outside-In causes you to say things to yourself such as "I know exercise is good for me. I should get out there and do something." "Why can't you get your lazy self over to the gym, you good-for-nothing sloth." "I have to lose weight before the summer so I can fit into my bathing suit." None of these statements will motivate you to exercise regularly, but I hear people say them all the time.

Without getting too bogged down in history and sociology, the main point is that Outside-In dominates our behavior because of the social, political, and economic structure of Western civilization. The main words guiding this structure are *rational* and *analytical*. We live in a society dominated by a rational view of life and people.

It's no wonder, then, that our mind listens to and at some level accepts much of the information about health and fit-

11

ness because it is based on research conducted from a rational, analytical perspective. It's everywhere — scientific journals, TV, magazines, newspapers. Whenever something is made rational, such as health and fitness, the focus is primarily on outcome: longevity, disease reduction, weight loss, and fitness.

This logic points us to the future: if we do this, then that should or will happen. Rationality focuses us on the desired products of exercise, but it moves us further away from any awareness and enjoyment of our exercise. The typical Outside-In approach completely ignores the fact that exercise is an *experience* and that people can be motivated — or not — by that experience.

Behavior change approaches such as educating yourself on the benefits of exercise, motivating yourself with rewards and incentives, and undergoing health screenings will largely fail. But exercise scientists keep trying to convince you. In 1995 a group of them published a host of physical activity guidelines in the *Journal of the American Medical Association*. They state, "Successfully changing our sedentary society into an active one will require effective dissemination and acceptance of the message that moderate physical activity confers health benefits." Although these guidelines are well intended, they come from the Outside-In approach. As Ken Goodrick, an associate professor at Baylor College of Medicine, says, "We know that if everybody exercised a few hours a week, Type 2 diabetes would be virtually nonexistent. The trick is motivating everyone to do it." There's no trick, really. It's just that as humans our behavior is not always rational. Before my wife and I gave up caffeine, there were times when we would drive the 45 minutes from our town to Cincinnati just to buy a cup of a certain brand of coffee. During the ride, we would tell each other how crazy we were being. We could have easily bought coffee in our own community, but the mental and emotional connection with the taste of the coffee available in Cincinnati made us do something that on a rational level seemed downright dumb. To change your behavior, you must tap into this deeper mental, emotional, and spiritual connection — what we sometimes call "irrational behavior." In essence, exercising regularly is irrational, and those who do it did not come to it solely by convincing themselves of all the wonderful, rational benefits.

Are You Tired of Hearing How Good Exercise Is for You?

In fact, only about one of five people exercise regularly, even though most people know about the health benefits of exercise and say they want to exercise.

When people are continually bombarded with Outside-In information, they begin to feel a helpless, mindless malaise toward moving their body. Or they get so desperate to "repair the damage" that they try things that are ineffective at best, unsafe at worst. Why else would some people take a pill before going to bed thinking that they will lose weight while they sleep? The Outside-In informational approach scares people, but they don't know how to find the key to their own motivation. So they turn to things that are just taking their money or feel guilty while doing nothing.

So don't feel too bad if you haven't been able to stay with a fitness program that you tried to follow in your newspaper or favorite magazine. Most of these approaches just spell out how to do the physical parts of exercise. For example, an article in *Cooking Light* magazine by Gin Miller, a fitness expert, laid out a 4-week program that included cardiovascular, strength, and flexibility components. She described how to do the exercises, when to do them, and so on. From a fitness perspective, the program seemed reasonable. Miller states, "The only thing you need to do is make time in your schedule and lace up your sneakers." The problem is, that's not the only thing, it's everything. You won't adhere to this kind of program without developing an inner reason for doing it. The how-to fitness information is certainly important, but changing your mindset is more important than any program. All programs begin and end, but your mind keeps going, and you'll need to change it if you want to keep moving your body.

Many fitness experts and programs almost unwittingly set people up for long-term failure. People already know the myriad benefits of regular exercise, yet they still can't motivate themselves to get moving. A survey conducted by American Sports Data tells us that 79 percent of the population already has a "highly developed fitness consciousness." Yet most people still fail to work exercise into their lives.

Even good exercise adherence programs tested by behavioral scientists come up a little short. Rod Dishman and Janet Buckworth at the University of Georgia analyzed the results of 127 studies designed to increase people's exercise behavior. People generally reverted to their earlier behavior shortly after most of the studies ended. Much of the scientific research has been successful only in getting people to exercise during the intervention. But the intervention has not been very effective in changing people's mindset. When typical Outside-In exercise programs are offered, 50 to 75 percent of the participants drop out within a few weeks or months.

Clearly, simply providing people with information doesn't work, and, in fact, overemphasizing the benefits of exercise can produce strong feelings of guilt, anxiety, and frustration, which result in even less motivation to exercise. Furthermore, people can become so focused on these outcomes that they ignore the process of developing positive, inner experiences with movement and exercise.

Telling people about all the benefits of exercise without helping them change their mindset toward the exercise is like putting children on a bike for the first time with no training wheels — they will crash.

Two Motivations for Exercise

Outside-In	Inside-Out
reduces disease risk	feels good
controls weight	enjoyable
future-oriented	in the present

Outside-In doesn't work. Becoming a regular exerciser has very little to do with your belief in the message that physical activity will enhance your long-term health. As you'll see, many people who do exercise regularly don't exercise primarily for a specific reason. It will take a lot more than your belief that accumulating 30 minutes of moderate physical activity is good for you to put in that time each day. Becoming a regular exerciser requires a transformation from an Outside-In focus to an Inside-Out experience. People who garden regularly don't do it because they think it's going to reduce their risk of coronary artery disease. They garden because they love the connection with the earth, the state of mind they enter when surrounded by flowers and greenery, the feelings of accomplishment derived from the aesthetics of the garden. These are powerful, inner reasons for gardening. Approaching exercise from an Inside-Out perspective will help you focus on the process and joy of your experience. Once you open up to that joy of movement, you'll want to do it more frequently. And if your life is anything like mine, you will need that inner force to inspire you to exercise while living in a chaotic time.

I Can't Exercise Because My Life Is Out of Control

Changes in family structure, advances in technology, and our work habits make it even less likely that an Outside-In approach will help people become regular exercisers. Women in particular face these issues. For example, single-parent households have increased significantly in the past 25 years, and most of these single parents are women who work. For all women, the pressures of juggling work and family are enormous.

More stress results from these changes, and stress has a negative effect on exercise. Barbara Stetson and her colleagues at the University of Louisville followed a group of women's exercise patterns for 8 weeks, examining their perceived stress each week and how it related to their behavior. Their findings showed that even minor stress, such as rushing to meet a deadline or completing household chores, severely disrupted the women's exercise patterns. When the perceived stress was the highest, the frequency of the women's exercise was the lowest. The researchers also found that under high stress, the women's confidence to achieve their exercise goal and enjoy exercise was diminished.

Suggesting that these women exercise for Outside-In reasons does nothing to ease those pressures, and it certainly does little to help them develop a passion or inner fire to move their bodies regardless of the barriers — such as time pressure — to exercise.

Other changes in family life have also had a major impact on people's leisure time. In 1960, only 40 percent of mothers with children from 6 to 17 were employed outside the home. By 1996, that figure had risen to 77 percent. As William Haskell of the Stanford University Center for Research in Disease Prevention points out, "Within households, much more time is spent working to earn a living in the 1990s than in the 1950s."

All of these changes have reduced people's leisure time,

not increased it, as some experts projected in the 1960s. This makes it more difficult for many people to perform healthy behaviors such as exercise. As Haskell writes,

> The expectation has been that we would be able to use new technology to accomplish a similar amount of work in less time and therefore increase the amount of leisure time available. Instead, we have used new technology to do more work in a similar amount of time, decreasing the amount of work-related physical activity but not making any additional time available for leisure activities.

Simply put, work rules. The downsizing phenomenon of the early 1990s left many people out of work. Many of them decided to start their own small businesses rather than return to corporate America. This is probably a good trend in the long run, but as anyone running a small business knows, it takes uncountable hours of blood, sweat, and tears. A national survey sponsored by Oxford Health Plans found that one in six American workers does not use up his or her annual vacation time due to job demands. What's more, since 1980, the number of workers who hold more than one job has risen by 54 percent. There are hardly enough hours in the day to fit in exercise with one job, let alone two.

The employees still in corporations now must do more with less — the lean and mean approach. So they work 10 to 12 hours a day instead of 8 or 9. And employers are reducing the average amount of vacation time for their workers. Some people commute as many as 2 hours to and from work each day. Unless they exercise at work or in place of lunch, when are they going to do it? Their commute can turn a 9-hour workday into a 13-hour workday. This barely leaves enough time at the end of the day to do anything but go to bed.

Paradoxically, the research on exercise in corporate settings shows that employees who are fit are absent less and more productive than inactive employees. Two reasons explain this phenomenon. Regular exercise strengthens your immune system, which helps you fight off illness, especially under high stress. So exercisers miss work less often. Also, research shows that spending too much time at one thing, such as work, fosters a mindless perspective — a lack of concentration.

Finding exercise solutions to these large barriers requires planning, organization, and an overwhelming desire to exercise. Most people don't have these skills and motivation, especially when no one is helping them develop those inner skills. You can understand why knowing about the benefits of exercise and actually exercising are two different things.

I want you to exercise regularly. You'll be happier and healthier, and in some way you'll make the world a better place. But know what you're up against. Awareness is the first step to changing your mindset toward exercise.

If You Develop the Right Mindset, You'll Make Time

Based on what is going on in the larger society and in people's lives, finding time to exercise does seem like a major barrier. Yet there are people who are able to exercise in spite of their harried lives. The results from exercise-adherence studies are very clear on this issue. First, in general, people who exercise regularly do not have more time on their hands than couch potatoes. Second, studies have shown that people who said they didn't exercise because their health and fitness center was too far or too hard to get to actually lived closer to exercise facilities than the regular attendees.

I certainly have problems finding time for exercise. My wife travels frequently, which leaves me as the primary caregiver for our children most of the week. If your day is anything like mine — kids, work, and daily hassles — you can see why it's so easy to throw in the exercise towel. A major point throughout this book is that the only way to overcome a life that works against physical activity is to develop powerful, positive Inside-Out thoughts and feelings related to your exercise. These powerful feelings will motivate you to exercise regularly. Your desire must be greater than the barriers. You have only a few windows of opportunity for exercise each day. If moving your body isn't a part of your mind, body, and soul, you won't do it. Of course, you could drastically change your lifestyle to give you more time to exercise. But that's highly unlikely. Instead, you must drastically change your views about when, how, and why you move your body. The good news is that developing a passion for exercise is possible. I've seen the Intrinsic Exerciser develop in people who previously thought regular exercisers were completely nuts.

The Need for the Inside-Out
Approach to Exercise

The result of the Outside-In approach, combined with people's inability to overcome powerful social barriers, is a society full of exercise wannabes with guilt complexes and high anxiety. In essence, it could be more unhealthy for you to know about the relationship between physical activity and long-term health than not knowing about it if you don't change your health habits.

The late Marshall Becker, a renowned medical sociologist at the University of Michigan, cited plenty of evidence in a classic article showing that the health and fitness movement has created a new segment of our population called "the worried well." They sit around worrying that they're not exercising enough, not eating a diet low in fat, and coping poorly with stress. They're not presently in any high-risk categories for disease but worry that they soon will be. So they think about all of the health behaviors, like exercise, that they should be doing, but most don't act on that worry. Those that do initiate some kind of change revert back to their old ways in a matter of months.

If you become more mindful of your exercise experience, you have a better chance of enjoying moving your body and in the process becoming an Intrinsic Exerciser, which you need to be to overcome the barriers to regular exercise described earlier. James Maddux of George Mason University hits the mark when he writes, "The secret to getting people to not only begin exercise routines but also to maintain them is to teach them to do it mindfully, to be in the present moment while doing it, to view exercise as something that is done for its own sake instead of for some future gain, to see exercise not as a struggle with death but instead as a celebration of life."

The route to celebrating life through exercise is an inner one, and that's what we'll begin to work on from the inside out.

2

....

Inside-Out: The Intrinsic Approach to Exercise

> Change — real change — comes from
> the inside out.
>
> — Stephen Covey, *The 7 Habits of*
> *Highly Effective People*

Let's say that the Outside-In approach, the extrinsic mindset toward exercise, has been relatively ineffective for you. That is, your exercise comes and goes like the tide no matter which program you try. Your next question probably is "But what do I do now?" Answer: you become an Intrinsic Exerciser. As the figure on the next page shows you, you start making the transformation from Outside-In to Inside-Out. It's a more powerful approach to exercising regularly and is supported by evidence from a variety of sources. As you'll see throughout this book, many people who become regular exercisers have been able to make this shift in their

23

mindset. In this chapter, I help you understand better what on some level you already know — that we were all born to move, and move frequently. It's primarily our brain and our culture that get in the way of moving our body — and enjoying it. We can't control our culture day in and day out, but we can control our thoughts and feelings.

Motivational Mindset Shift

Extrinsic (product)	Intrinsic (process)
reduce risk of disease	feels good
control/lose weight	enjoyment (flow)
enhanced fitness	mastery
future	present
have to	want to

MINDSET SHIFT IS CRITICAL FOR
LONG-TERM BEHAVIOR CHANGE

Examples of an intrinsic mindset for exercise are all over the place if you pay attention and take the inner path. Laura Fraser, a regular exerciser, wrote in *Mode* about how she applies the benefits of intrinsic motivation in her own way: "I couldn't care less about the goal; what I like is the process. I like the sensation of walking outside in the fresh air, soaring down a hill on my bicycle, dancing up a sweat, swimming meditative laps." Bill Rodgers, the world's premier marathoner two decades ago, who still runs, says in a *Sports Illustrated* interview, "I believe in living an active life — using your body and your muscles. We're all meant to move. We're all meant to be athletes." He's right. You were meant to move — and it started thousands of years ago.

The Origins of the Intrinsic Exerciser

Nigel Nicholson, a professor of organizational behavior at London Business School, writes that "you can take the person out of the Stone Age, but you can't take the Stone Age out of the person." Our Stone Age ancestors were physically active. Some evolutionary psychologists would suggest that we are hard-wired for movement, living in a body that wants to move. It's only our present society and culture that have shifted us away from our moving roots.

Writing in the *Journal of Human Evolution*, Walter Bortz, M.D., presents a compelling argument that early humans were extremely active. About 5 million years ago, our evolutionary branch split from that of the great apes. The two major behavioral departures from those relatively static creatures seem to be the introduction of a high proportion of meat in the diet and *a high level of sustained physical activity*. Bortz writes, "These changes constitute a positive feedback loop which is self-perpetuating. These two features, mutually complementary, are proposed to have contributed substantially to the two major discriminatory characters of *Homo sapiens*, our brains and our adaptability."

Our brains have evolved partly because we have been physically active over thousands of years. And we're not just talking about our ancestors here. More recent research published by scientists from the Salk Institute for Biological Studies in La Jolla, California, has shown that activity levels significantly influence our brain. Their work shows that some physical activities promote the growth of new neurons while measurably prolonging the survival of existing brain cells. The researchers found that adult mice exercising on running wheels regularly developed twice as many new brain cells in the hippocampus portion of the brain as mice housed in standard cages. The hippocampus plays a role in our memory of new facts and events. More recently, these researchers even found this process occurred in older adults.

Fred Gage, the senior author of the Salk study, suggests that physical activity prompts the nervous system to prepare for an onslaught of new information the way an animal navigates unfamiliar terrain in the pursuit of prey or in flight from an enemy. As Bernd Heinrich, a professor of biology at the University of Vermont, writes, "Our abilities to run, throw, and jump are leftovers in our survival tool kits. As such, we use them in play because they are instinctually important to us." What's more, the research of Steven Reiss, a professor of psychology and psychiatry at Ohio State University, suggests that physical activity is one of the sixteen basic desires of happiness.

I sometimes hear from sedentary people who think that exercise is just not inside them. They then give up on themselves, thinking that they cannot perform regular exercise. They are wrong, for everybody is wired for regular physical activity. Exercise has been instrumental in the development of our brains and in our capacity to adapt to our environment. Some 99 percent of the time that humans have existed has been spent as a physically active population. It is only in the more recent 1 percent — time spent as farmers, as assembly line workers, and as information technicians — that we have become physically inactive.

We were born to move. So if you aren't active on a regular basis, you can't achieve your true potential. I have spent some time on this point to demonstrate that the motivation and the inclination to be physically active are there for each of us. As the University of Utah exercise physiologist Pat Eisenman points out, "We are biologically equipped for one kind of lifestyle, but forced by cultural circumstances to live another."

So the main challenge for most of us is to find the Intrinsic Exerciser that lies within. Of course, this is not an easy challenge. But every time you think of reasons not to exercise, say: I WAS BORN TO MOVE. BY MOVING REGULARLY, I WILL MOVE CLOSER TO BECOMING WHO I WAS MEANT TO BE.

Born to Move

A basic psychological or motivational component of this inner desire to move is called *intrinsic motivation.*

The late Robert White, a psychologist at Harvard, proposed in 1959 that we are all born with a desire to have an effect on things. As children, we naturally explore our environment. I can still remember when my son was about 18 months old, he would continually drop his food from the highchair onto the floor to see what would happen. This is really the first inkling of intrinsic motivation. We start off doing things because novelty and curiosity motivate us.

Watching toddlers play, we can see that many times they are motivated by no other reason than the play itself. Of course, child development experts explain that this play is very important for a child's development. These are all positive outcomes of the child's play. They are doing the play for its own sake.

As we grow older, our experiences with other people, school, and more can begin to squelch this innate desire to do things simply because we want to. We are taught to do many things as a means to an end. Do well on your test scores so you can get into college; do your homework so that you can do well on the test; practice your sport so you can get an athletic scholarship; exercise so you can lose weight. We tie extrinsic outcomes to our actions.

I've heard several versions of this story over the years.

I used to live in a house with a big, grassy yard across the street. I loved sitting on the porch in the evening and staring out into the peacefulness of that yard. It wasn't mine but felt like it was. Then one day neighborhood kids started playing in the field. They were so loud and noisy, they were ruining my evening peace. I tried yelling at them to please go play somewhere else, but that only made it worse. So I devised a plan to get rid of them.

I walked to that yard one day and told the children I had changed my mind and actually enjoyed their playing so much that I would give them each a quarter if they would keep playing in the yard each evening. I did that for about one week. I could tell they were pleased as punch for taking money when they already loved to play on the site. After a week, I told them I was running out of money and could only give each one a dime. After another week, I said I could only afford a nickel. There was some hemming and hawing, but they still came. A week later I walked over one more time and said, "I'm sorry, but I'm so low on money, all I can afford is a penny for each of you." They all looked at me as if I were nuts and said, "Forget you, we're not going to come play here for a lousy penny. We're going somewhere else." And they did.

The story clearly illustrates the different actions motivated by Outside-In and Inside-Out. The children went from being intrinsically motivated to play in the field to tying their play to an extrinsic reward. When the reward was taken away, their intrinsic motivation no longer existed, so it was no longer fun to play in the field. Does that sound familiar? When we are young, we love to learn to write our name, to read, to pretend. Then we get to school (grades become rewards), then go to work (money becomes the reward), and we end up working primarily for extrinsic reasons. The same thing can happen to our physical activity.

White also suggests that physical activity is a basic psychological need. He argues that physical activity is the foundation of all cognitive development. He cites one study — with rats, of course — showing that they would run in an activity wheel to an extent that could be correlated with their previous degree of confinement. They seemed to want to run, he writes, and they continued to run for such long times that no part of the behavior could readily be singled out as a consummatory response. Aren't there days when you feel like a rat, sitting in your office, confined indoors? Don't you ever get an urge just to be free and move your body in some way? I get them all the time. These are signals that your body wants to move. You only have to start listening to these signals and then act on them.

Intrinsic Motivation

Findings from myriad studies on exercise adherence show that people who have an intrinsic orientation for exercise have a good experience and exercise frequently. Put another way, exercise for intrinsic reasons and you will exercise more and enjoy it more. If you really want to exercise regularly, you'll need to develop an Intrinsic Exerciser mindset. Len Wankel at the University of Alberta published a study based on interviews of both maintainers and dropouts of an exercise program. He found that they all started for extrinsic reasons — anticipated health benefits or outcomes. Yet the maintainers were the ones who concentrated more on the intrinsic — things like mastery, learning, curiosity, and enjoyment — to help motivate themselves on the path to regular exercise.

Consider this chart describing the continuum for motivation:

No Motivation	Extrinsic Motivation				Intrinsic Motivation		
not motivated at all	external control	internal pressure	identified regulation	integrated regulation	to know	accomplishment	stimulation

"No motivation" is not you unless you have so much money that you just throw it away on exercise books. Extrinsic motivation actually comprises four different kinds of motivation. The first, external control, means that your exercise behavior is motivated or regulated through external means, such as rewards or your physician telling you that you need to lose some weight. Next is internal pressure. With this form of extrinsic motivation, you replace the external control with your own internal control. You now believe in the benefits of exercise and keep telling yourself, "I should exercise" or "I have to exercise." The third type is identified regulation. You can exercise sometimes just through sheer willpower, but you don't like it. You choose to do it, but you probably wouldn't unless you didn't have a lot of self-discipline. This is the approach that some talk show hosts recommend — just do it, even if it's not fun. People stuck in identified regulation look to personal trainers to help them get through it. I'm not against personal trainers, but they're expensive over a long period of time and they can unwittingly keep your mindset in the extrinsic zone. The final form of extrinsic motivation is integrated regulation, which is getting you close to the mindset shift for exercising for intrinsic reasons. You see and feel that the behavior is becoming a part of who you are. You're still not doing the activity for its own sake, but you are far removed from external and internal pressures.

Motivational scientists also suggest that there are three kinds of intrinsic motivation. *Exercising to know* means that you're engaging in exercise for the pleasure and satisfaction you experience while learning something new. Exercise is a wonderful way to explore aspects of others as well as yourself. A new aerobics class can teach you a lot about your body and your mind.

Exercising toward accomplishments means you are exercising for the pleasure and satisfaction experienced while you are challenging yourself or accomplishing something. Many nonexercisers train for a marathon as a means of challenging themselves to accomplish something they haven't done before. They then become regular exercisers and move on to the next accomplishment: perhaps lowering their time in the next marathon. This may seem somewhat extrinsic, but the point is that these people are striving for outcomes or goals. The primary source of motivation comes from the striving and the challenge.

Exercising to experience stimulation means you want pleasant feelings associated mainly with your senses — touching, seeing, hearing, smelling, and tasting. Many exercisers actually love the feeling of doing yoga, love the smell of sweat during an aerobics class. When pumping iron, some exercisers love the feel of their muscles working.

To know, to accomplish, and to experience stimulation are all different forms of intrinsic motivation, meaning you are motivated to exercise primarily for the pleasure and satisfaction of the experience itself. The experience connects with who you are. There is a high level of self-determination before, during, and after these exercise sessions.

A radio program asked a personal trainer to describe what happens to attendance at her facility in February compared with that in January. She said that three quarters of the people who showed up in January did not come the following month. The dropouts need to make a commitment, she said. They say they don't have time, but hey, we open at 5:00 A.M. Unfortunately, the personal trainer did not help people develop the inner fire to move their bodies. People who are focused on extrinsic motivation don't know how to make a commitment.

Here is a quiz to suggest where you might be right now on the motivation continuum for exercise. Place a check next to the single item that best describes your motivation for exercise (check only one). Be honest with yourself.

WHY ARE YOU CURRENTLY PARTICIPATING IN EXERCISE? OR WHY WOULD YOU PARTICIPATE IN EXERCISE IF NOT CURRENTLY DOING SO?

- ❏ 1. For the satisfaction it gives me to increase my knowledge about the activity.

- ❏ 2. Because I feel pressure from others to participate.

- ❏ 3. Because I feel I have to do it.

- ❏ 4. Because I think that exercise allows me to feel better about myself.

- ❏ 5. Because it is consistent with what I value.

- ❏ 6. For the pleasure of mastering the activity.

- ❏ 7. For the satisfaction I feel when I get into the flow of the activity.

- ❏ 8. I have no idea.

ANSWERS:

1. Intrinsic — to know.
2. Extrinsic — external control.
3. Extrinsic — internal pressure.

4. Extrinsic — identified regulation.
5. Extrinsic — integrated regulation.
6. Intrinsic — to accomplish.
7. Intrinsic — to experience stimulation.
8. No motivation.

Numbers 1, 6, and 7 are all forms of exercising for intrinsic reasons. If you checked any of these answers, you have the potential to experience a high level of intrinsic motivation toward your exercise.

Numbers 2, 3, 4, and 5 are forms of exercising for extrinsic reasons. If you checked any of these answers, you are probably experiencing low levels of intrinsic motivation toward your exercise.

Number 8 is a form of no motivation. If you checked it, you are experiencing very low levels of both intrinsic and extrinsic motivation toward your exercise.

Science Supports the Intrinsic Exerciser

A study at the University of Texas run by Laura Field and Mary Steinhardt showed that people who exercise primarily for enjoyment have higher physical self-esteem than people who focus on the outcomes and rewards of exercise. And if you feel good about your body, you'll be more likely to keep an exercise program going. Research conducted by Deborah Kendzierski and Kenneth DeCarlo at Villanova University used what they call the Physical Activity Enjoyment Scale to examine the link between exercise and enjoyment. The scale includes primarily intrinsic items. Results showed that the study participants chose to perform an activity and worked harder when they enjoyed it. Overall, Inside-Out is the most effective way to motivate yourself to exercise regularly. Research from the Canadian

Fitness and Lifestyle Research Institute, reported by the YMCA of Canada, says that regular exercisers claim that the best sources of motivation are

- fun, enjoyment, stimulation
- a feeling of accomplishment
- the pleasure of learning
- a concrete benefit, such as sleeping better and feeling calmer.

You can see how three of these four sources are closely aligned with the three components of intrinsic motivation — to know, to accomplish, to experience stimulation.

The Intrinsic Mindset Is Not Just a Scientific Fabrication

If I can't convince you with science, I'll persuade you with examples and the intrinsic philosophies of real people, people who have become Intrinsic Exercisers.

In *How to Feel Great 24 Hours a Day*, the late running philosopher George Sheehan writes about the mindset shift that occurs when going from a beginning exerciser to one who does it consistently over a long period of time. He used the words *Jogger*, *Runner*, and *Racer* as metaphors for the different mindsets. The *Jogger* mindset is similar to my Outside-In notion: the jogger focuses on the physical benefits — weight loss, longevity, reduction in risk of disease. But Sheehan says, "The fact is that few people will exercise for any length of time without the additional motives of both play and sport." Sheehan uses the *Runner* mindset as a metaphor for play and the *Racer* mindset as a metaphor for sport. They are both essential to motivating yourself to exercise and move you beyond a Jogger mentality.

The mind of a Runner focuses on the playlike aspects of exercise. Sheehan writes, "Play returns us to childhood. It allows complete freedom. Play is unstructured and without rules. It liberates us from necessity. It asks no product, no particular performance. It refuses to be serious. Play opens up our inner world and allows our subconscious to percolate through to understanding." By viewing your exercise as play, Sheehan believes, you will unlock emotion, understanding, and creativity that you never thought possible. The meaning of the exercise experience will be greatly enhanced.

The Racer mentality is different in that it moves you into a competitive realm. Sheehan is not talking about your becoming an elite athlete. All he's suggesting is that in a sport mode, you are more likely to challenge your physical and psychological limits. He argues that this approach is very motivating, that "sport makes us fully functioning adults. Through pushing to our limits, we grow in self-esteem and self-respect." And the nice thing is that you can adopt this approach without comparing yourself with other people. You can challenge yourself and your body in a variety of ways without worrying about what other people are doing.

When you have a chance, watch a five-minute scene in *Forrest Gump* that shows how the main character started exercising. The beginning of the scene shows him sitting in a chair on his front stoop, deep in thought. Then Gump's narrative voice says, "That day, for no particular reason, I decided to go for a little run." The subsequent segments show him running across the country and back. He just keeps going. The media, of course, keep asking him why he's doing it. For world hunger? For peace? The character replies, "I just felt like running." Sheehan and Forrest Gump both realize that the reasons for exercising are relatively simple, inner ones. Consider a childhood experience of mine. When I was 11 or 12, I rode my stingray bike into town and back home with my brother every day in the summer months. We rode the mile and a half into town to play with other kids at the Parks and Recreation Center. We lived at the crest of a long, gradual hill, and my brother and I would have coasting contests down the hill into town. What a blast: that was a feeling of complete freedom. We were totally absorbed in the moment, trying to hang on as long as possible without pedaling. We never thought about the difficulty of the return trip.

As we get older, we often think too far ahead. We think about how hard something will be or the consequences of our actions. Or we think of all the good and bad outcomes of a possible course of action, or whether we can do it or not, instead of just jumping right in.

Youth Sport: Outside-In in Disguise?

Surveys show that more kids are participating in organized youth sports — such as soccer and basketball — than ever before. Many are getting a good chunk of their physical activity when they are practicing these sports. Youth sport has a lot of good intentions and can have many positive effects.

But I think there's a danger, in that it leads to a lot of lazy kids and is partly responsible for this generation of children's low physical activity and fitness levels. Even worse, youth sport could be detracting from the number of kids who will want to participate in regular exercise as adults.

In youth sport, almost everything the children do is determined by an outside source. Times for playing are determined by practices and games; the amount of time a child plays is determined by the coach; where a child plays is determined by his or her ability and the coach. Success is based on extrinsic outcomes (won or lost), and trophies and awards are doled out accordingly. Children can believe that the only time to be physically active is when an adult tells them to or when there is some extrinsic reason for it.

Once children's physical activity gets tied to extrinsic motivation, what do they do when those external forces are gone? Nothing! We call this laziness, but what has really happened is that their intrinsic motivation has been undermined by their youth sport experience. This leads to kids who have no ability or desire to initiate their own physical activity. They don't know how. That's why so many adults say, "Kids don't want to do anything anymore," and why many kids say, "I'm bored. I don't know what to do." Well, it's not their fault but that of adults who are obsessed with overorganizing children's physical activity within an Outside-In philosophy.

When I look back on my own sport experiences, I begin to see that everything I did from the time I was to born to about age 12 prepared me to direct my own physical activity experiences internally more than 30 years later. I'm now so glad that my friends and I organized our own activities, to which we gave names such as barn basketball, mud football, onion field whiffleball, sock 'em soccer, pickle ball, infield, and over-the-roof softball.

I was building a powerful base of intrinsic motivation and problem solving through these activities. I was involved in the whole process of making rules, deciding when and where we were going to play, calling plays in the huddle, strategizing with my teammates, and determining when to quit. In an interview in *People*, Dr. Richard Strauss, the director of the childhood weight control program at the Robert Wood Johnson Medical School in New Brunswick, New Jersey, voices his concern about our children's physical activity. He and his colleagues conducted a study that showed, on average, children spend *only 12 minutes a day* running or playing hard. He's convinced this lack of physical activity has led to dramatic increases in childhood obesity. He writes, "I believe that unless a child learns to *enjoy* [emphasis added] vegetables, fruits, whole grain foods and physical activity, little can be done."

Children are not being taught, through youth sport or much else, how to enjoy or direct their own physical activity. Because of my internally directed experiences as a child, I believe that it was easier for me to begin and maintain exercise as an adult. I had the inner motivation, the skills, and the problem-solving capabilities that are needed.

We need to combat the extrinsic orientation of youth

39

sport by limiting the amount of time children participate in activities organized by adults. We then need to provide them with many opportunities for controlling and directing their own physical activity. Children already know how to do this to some extent; we just need to nudge them a little and then get out of the way. If we don't, we are going to have a generation of children who become the next generation of sedentary adults.

Preparing for the Less Traveled, Inner Exercise Road

I realize that the notion of mindset transformation about exercise may be new to you. But I think it's quite clear that as we get older and more set in the system, many of us are guided by extrinsic motivation in our daily life. Mihaly Csikszentmihalyi, a psychologist at Claremont Graduate School in Claremont, California, suggests that many individuals experience their day "as drudgery to be endured only for the sake of future rewards." This isn't a very enjoyable way to live, but many people accept it.

But we can make a conscious choice about being active or sedentary. Exercise is a voluntary behavior. People can choose whether to do it or not without any immediate, negative consequences. Once you begin to approach exercise in an intrinsic way, you'll enjoy it and naturally move your body more frequently — and you'll reap the benefits of weight control, a possible reduction in the risk of disease, and a longer life.

3
....

The Intrinsic Exerciser:
An Overview

> One is alive when and because one moves,
> but totally alive when the movements are
> spontaneous, vital, alive, and free.
>
> — Brian Fahey, *The Passionate Body*

To become an Intrinsic Exerciser, you begin to transform your way of thinking and feeling about exercise. You begin to *experience* exercise rather than just going through the physical motions. I have identified four components of the Intrinsic Exerciser mindset:

- Vision
- Mastery
- Flow
- Inergy

Each component is an innate, natural part of who we are.

Vision

The first step is *vision*. Humans have the innate ability to see into the future. Heinrich writes, "We have the unique ability to keep in mind what is not before the eye . . . Human beings with the longest vision tend to make the biggest mark. Vision allows us to reach into the future."

For example, vision is a critical part of most self-help development books, although it is rarely applied to health behavior or exercise behavior change. To become an Intrinsic Exerciser, you must use your innate ability to visualize yourself as an exerciser without actually exercising. The vision begins to make exercise personally meaningful, which starts the mindset transformation process.

What does it mean to apply vision to your exercise? It means you use exercise to explore who you are, to articulate why you are exercising and what you hope to get from it. You must look ahead and envision yourself as a regular exerciser. A clear vision creates your desire, your passion to move your body on a regular basis. Notice that this kind of vision has nothing to do with long-range Outside-In goals, such as losing weight or reducing your risk of disease. You have to be a mover first. Your vision must connect to how you want to feel about your exercise before, during, and after you do it.

To develop this vision, you start working on the image you have of your present and your future physical self. The point here is that you must activate what Hazel Markus, a psychologist at Stanford University, calls a *possible self* with respect to moving your body. You must see and feel yourself exercising before you actually do it. Top athletes do this all the time: they see themselves exercising and performing at their very peak. You can do this too, and it begins to make exercise personally meaningful to you. It also enhances self-awareness.

Mastery

As you develop your own vision for how you want to experience exercise, you begin to work on *mastery*. With mastery you draw on your natural desire to improve, to grow. You learn to focus on your own performance by setting goals that parallel the three aspects of intrinsic motivation — to know, accomplish, stimulate.

With a mastery focus you can be successful no matter what's going on around you. In fact, an essential characteristic of mastery is that you base success on your own criteria. Your goals are always related to the exercise itself, not to the outcomes or the environment. You don't compare your physical ability or performance with that of other people. Rather, you challenge yourself during the workout — lift 5 more pounds, walk 5 more minutes. Your goal on one day can be to walk fast; on another day it can be to walk slowly and focus on your surroundings.

Mastery helps you become immune to changes in your environment. You develop the mindset to exercise under any conditions — good or bad. Mastery is Inside-Out because you base your success solely on your own criteria; you are in control of your goals and success, which is what being intrinsically motivated is all about. This doesn't mean that you never compete; some exercisers love to compete. The point, however, is that with a mastery focus you use competition to help you achieve your own goals.

Flow

The third part of becoming an Intrinsic Exerciser is flow, which Csikszentmihalyi has defined as an optimal psychological state involving total absorption in and connection to an activity. With flow, your exercise leaves you with a feeling of satisfaction. Staying in the moment during each and every exercise session is what flow is all about.

Similar to vision and mastery, flow or optimal experience is a vital part of being human. Fausto Massimini, Csikszentmihalyi, and Antonella Delle Fave at the University of Milan Medical School write, "Clearly, enjoyment is the main reason for the selection and retention of most artistic cultural forms. Painting, music, drama, and even the mere ability to write are symbolic skills adopted because they produce positive states of consciousness." For movement and physical activity to remain part of our culture, they need to be driven by enjoyment. For you to participate in exercise regularly, you need some flow experiences.

Individuals in flow are concentrating on the task at hand and not easily distracted. The idea is simple: flow experiences help you enjoy the activity so much that you want to perform it for its own sake and will go to great lengths to do so. Csikszentmihalyi describes this as an "autotelic experience," one that is intrinsically rewarding. Statements such as "I was on a high" and "I totally lost track of time" illustrate people's typical descriptions of a flow experience. When you stretch your physical capacity, integrate your mind and body, and fully immerse yourself in the activity, the outcome is likely to provide powerful intrinsic rewards. As an Intrinsic Exerciser, you experience flow in your physical activity, and that's what draws you back to it.

Flow can help you create a very strong mental and emotional bond with moving your body. Attaining a flow experience, at least some of the time, will help motivate you to exercise when most people come up with reasons not to. And achieving it can be easier than you think. The science of flow shows that it can occur in any activity and that the actor, player, or exerciser has a great deal of control and choice over the mental state attained.

Flow also generates positive emotions, helps you control the experience, keeps you from boredom and anxiety, builds concentration and attention skills, and develops the "for its own sake" attitude.

Inergy

The last step is what I call *Inergy* — energy that comes from the inside out. Inergy is about making connections among your mind, body, and spirit. It's based on the science and philosophy of wellness, which is all about humans striving to be whole. Wellness theory suggests that we all have needs that must be balanced and integrated to achieve optimal functioning and well-being. Striving for wellness or the integration of your needs is as natural as a baby's learning to walk. This is why Inergy fits the Intrinsic Exerciser idea. The whole point is to tap into what is natural about who you are and who you want to become. The Intrinsic Exerciser helps to push you along an inner path that in some sense you already understand as it relates to moving your body. The Intrinsic Exerciser helps you awaken the connections among your body, mind, and spirit and to show you that a life without movement isn't really living. As Alfred Adler once wrote, "There can no longer be any doubt today that everything we call a body shows a striving to become whole."

Again, Inergy, like vision, mastery, and flow, is a natural part of who we are. Wellness is all about the whole being greater than the sum of its parts. It's not just about balancing your needs or indulging in one need — it's about bringing them together. That's when the oneness, the wholeness, occurs. That's where optimal functioning occurs as well as learning and personal development. As you will see, the idea with Inergy in the context of the Intrinsic Exerciser is *to synergize, connect, integrate your physical need with your other needs, mental, social, and spiritual.* Through Inergy, you will create the last link in a powerful inner, motivational chain that will spur you on — fuel the fire — to move your body on a regular basis. Viewed in this way, you can begin to transform yourself into an Intrinsic Exerciser by paying closer attention to how your physical activity spills over into or meshes with your other needs. In fact, you plan and structure many of your exercise experiences so that you optimize the opportunities for Inergy. In essence, you consciously plan for Inergy.

Inergy helps you maintain the passion for exercise that you have started with vision, mastery, and flow.

On Becoming an Intrinsic Exerciser

To optimize your Intrinsic Exerciser mindset — vision, mastery, flow, and Inergy — you'll want to combine the four components as much as possible so together they can reshape your attitudes and experiences with exercise.

The first two steps — vision and mastery — get you to move your body. In essence, they activate and focus your mind on how to begin changing your behavior from the inside out. These two steps are the catalysts of action; they create an inner desire for you to begin moving. Vision helps you begin to feel like an exerciser; mastery helps you know what it's like to be a successful exerciser.

The last two steps — flow and Inergy — keep you connected to the joyful inner experience of moving your body on a regular basis. Flow keeps you in the moment to optimize every exercise experience; Inergy helps you connect exercise with your other needs. Flow provides the enjoyment in the moment; Inergy keeps you going.

Combined, these four steps provide a powerful inner motivational system for becoming an intrinsic, regular exerciser for the rest of your life, no matter the circumstances.

Intrinsic Exercisers focus on how much fun they're having and how good they feel about themselves when they move their bodies. Everyone should be able to feel like this. It's not a secret: by working through the simple exercises in this book and learning to incorporate the four steps, anyone can become a regular exerciser.

What follows is the Intrinsic Exerciser Self-Assessment. This is not a scientific instrument nor a test. But it should give you a good idea of where you are in terms of experiencing exercise in an intrinsic way. I like to record my assessment every few months just to see how my intrinsic mindset is doing. You may want to take this assessment again after you have put into practice some of the Intrinsic Exerciser strategies I'm about to share.

INTRINSIC EXERCISER SELF-ASSESSMENT

1. The main point to moving my body is to experience it in the here and now. ❑ Agree ❑ Disagree

2. Moving my body is not about long-term outcomes but about the experience. ❑ Agree ❑ Disagree

3. When I move my body I feel free. ❑ Agree ❑ Disagree

4. I experience my movement without judging my body. ❑ Agree ❑ Disagree

5. When I move my body, I forget about thinking and let my senses (feel, smell, taste, touch, hearing) take over. ❑ Agree ❑ Disagree

6. I allow my movement to embrace my whole being — mind, body, and spirit. ❑ Agree ❑ Disagree

7. I am aware of my basic bodily signals and my bodily tension hot points. ❑ Agree ❑ Disagree

8. I am aware of my breathing and how it varies through different movements. ❑ Agree ❑ Disagree

9. I regularly distract my mind from my body during movement experiences. ❑ Agree ❑ Disagree

10. I can focus on one thought or one feeling for at least 5 minutes during a movement activity. ❑ Agree ❑ Disagree

11. I perform exercise as a mindful experience rather than as a mindless habit. ❑ Agree ❑ Disagree

12. I often worry that others are evaluating my body when I am moving. ❑ Agree ❑ Disagree

13. I sometimes connect exercise with my need to interact with others (social). ❑ Agree ❑ Disagree

14. I sometimes connect exercise with my need to learn (mental). ❑ Agree ❑ Disagree

15. I sometimes connect exercise with my need for meaning and purpose (spiritual). ❑ Agree ❑ Disagree

Scoring: Give yourself 1 point for "Agree" responses except for numbers 9 and 12. For those numbers give yourself 1 point if you responded "Disagree."

Totals:

12–15: You are well on your way to becoming an Intrinsic Exerciser. This book will enhance the process.

8–11: You have the makings of an Intrinsic Exerciser. Dig in on the strategies in this book to help you become the ultimate Intrinsic Exerciser.

4–7: The Intrinsic Exerciser is in there somewhere. This book will help you find it.

0–3: Your inner exercise tank is on empty. Let's start filling it up.

Part II

Four Steps to Developing the Intrinsic Exerciser Mindset

4
....

Step 1: Activate the Intrinsic Exerciser with Vision

> What we can do, and only we can do it (a machine cannot), is create a new behavior.
>
> — William Glasser, *The Quality School*

Mary was a good athlete when she was younger, but after having two children and performing a demanding sales job, she doesn't recognize her body anymore. She knows she needs to exercise, but it's been about five years since she "made up her mind" to do it, but she has not been able to get back into it on a regular basis. She bought some kick-boxing videotapes (used once; her kids ask her what those boxing tapes are for under the TV), purchased an exercise bike (used twice; her kids use the heart rate monitor to lasso Buzz Lightycar), joined the health club in town (went twice, just to see if that new personal trainer she heard about might be able to help her), and visited a spa for a week (very pleasant, but expensive, massages). Yet her exercise behavior remains the same as it was five years ago — sporadic. Mary is an excellent professional who doesn't consider herself lazy or unmotivated. She can't quite figure out what's going on. She's still a young woman and wants to get her exercise act together.

Mary, like millions of other women and men, has made the cardinal sin of focusing on technical, or Outside-In, products and services first as the way to develop an exercise routine. Perhaps you're making the same mistake right now. If so, STOP! You know deep down that these Outside-In things aren't going to work. Your intrinsic tank is on empty, and that's the only thing that's going to drive you to move. So your first step is to fill up that empty tank with personal meaning and a passion for exercise. You do that by activating your vision. Spending some time to create a meaningful vision of yourself as an exerciser doesn't cost $50 for 30 minutes with a personal trainer. Doing some mindset shifting — from Outside-In to Inside-Out — is free and will help you develop the inner passion for moving your body, to awaken the mover within.

20/20 Exercise Vision

The vision step has two parts: a *physical vision* and an *inner vision*. Intrinsic Exercisers have 20/20 vision; they can see themselves clearly as exercisers (physical vision) even when they are inactive and they know how they want their exercise to make them feel (inner vision). *Physical vision is all about the kind of exerciser you want to become; inner vision is how you want your exercise to feel.* Both are important to your becoming a regular exerciser. Your goal as an Intrinsic Exerciser is to begin to activate your inner path to movement through the creation of both an image of self that includes exercise and an inner image of the positive feelings that exercise can give you.

To develop physical and inner vision is not difficult, but most people who try to exercise do not work on either one. They think they do, but they don't. Their take on outer vision is to lose 20 pounds. That's not vision. That's a goal. And most people don't really know how they want their exercise to feel. Vision begins successful exercise behavior change.

I'll give you an example. My wife, Kim, was once at a conference for a few days. On Monday afternoon our son, Colin, got sick. The next day was supposed to be an exercise day for me. I was primed. Gearing up for the Heart Mini-Marathon, I was looking forward to a longer run. But I had to stay home with Colin. In the back of my mind throughout the day I was thinking about a way to run. As the day went on, Colin started to feel better, so I called Chris, who provides day care for him, and asked if I could bring him over at the day's end so I could get a run in. She agreed. I ran, felt better, raised my energy, and was home alone with both of my children that evening.

I tell this story to show that my vision for myself as an

exerciser, as a runner, is clear and strong. My physical vision is that I can see myself exercising, I can see that it's possible, it's part of who I am. And my inner vision is all about the feelings of being strong, having energy, enjoying physical accomplishment. This 20/20 vision pulls me toward movement. I figure out a way. Then, once I'm moving, I experience exercise in such a way that it affirms my vision — not to mention mastery, flow, and Inergy, which I'll get to in the next few chapters. Without vision, you won't seize the exercise day. You'll retreat from the barriers of the day and give up.

No Limits with Physical Vision

Physical vision is all about how you see your physical self in the future. The great thing about being human is that we all have the ability to see ourselves differently in the future. You may not be an exerciser today, but you can see yourself as an exerciser tomorrow or the next day. And how we see ourselves in the future determines how we behave now, tomorrow, and the next day. Robert Sonstroem, an educational psychologist, writes, "We tend to act as our conception of self dictates to us." Along with Paul Nurius, Markus writes, "Possible selves are the ideal selves we would very much like to become." She explains that unless you have a strong vision of the self you want to be, your behavior will not change no matter how hard you try. For our purposes, I'm calling Markus's notion of possible selves "physical vision." The main point is that you must develop a vision, a possible exercise self, to get you on the inner path to behavior change.

Now, here's the beauty of physical vision and why it's part of the Intrinsic Exerciser: you control what self you become. What you are not now, you can become if you can see it in your mind's eye and feel it in your gut. If you begin to visualize yourself as someone who exercises, your behavior will start to match that vision because you will be more aware of the movement possibilities.

Think about the process of buying a new car. For years, we owned a Honda Accord and we would see other Accords all over the place. Then, with the arrival of our children, we started to think about a van. We saw ourselves driving a van with the whole family. Once this possibility was in our consciousness, we started to see vans everywhere. This is called selective attention. Once you imbed in your consciousness the vision of yourself as an exerciser, you will exercise more simply because you will become more aware of your body and movement. Csikszentmihalyi writes, "If the self includes everything that passes in consciousness, it follows that what we pay attention to over time will shape the self."

It goes both ways: a clear physical vision of a possible exercise self begins to help you pay attention, and paying attention and being more aware helps to shape and strengthen the vision. Research with possible selves supports this notion. A study of older adults by Karen Hooker of Syracuse University and Cheryl Kaus of the State University of New York at Oswego found that those who had indicated a strong hoped-for self in the area of health participated in more health-promoting behaviors, such as exercise, than those adults who didn't see themselves behaving in healthful practices. A study by Deborah Kendzierski at Villanova University showed that college students who viewed themselves as exercisers, even though they weren't presently exercising, were more likely to start an exercise program at a future time than those students who saw themselves as nonexercisers.

Developing a possible exercise self is not just an exercise in positive thinking. It goes way beyond that. Positive thinking about exercising won't do any good unless it's connected to a vision you have of yourself as an exerciser. In that case, you will pay attention to the things that will help you exercise more frequently.

Expunging the Extrinsic

Many people carry around an image of their body based on what they see, read, and hear. They then begin an exercise program based on a fuzzy notion of that information. There's no connection between the behavioral attempts and the physical self. The first thing to do is eliminate the images created by Outside-In or the extrinsic approach to exercise behavior change I described in Chapter 1. Starting right now, avoid or take less seriously any information that appears to be from Outside-In sources. I'm in complete agreement with the *Runner's World* columnist John Bingham, who writes,

Step 1: Activate the Intrinsic Exerciser with Vision

Of all the ways to succeed at failing, none has had a more profound impact on the American population's psyche than the diet and fitness industries. The success of these industries relies on failure. For them to be successful, we must fail. They must make *sure* that we fail. If we, the dollar-spending consumers, succeeded at dieting and getting into shape, the diet and fitness industries would disappear within a year.

Here are some ways to clear your mind to prepare for the new self or vision you will develop:

• Tune out the TV news, newspapers, infomercials, and radio. Don't watch infomercials relating to exercise equipment or videos. If one comes on and you can't find the remote, run as fast as you can out of the room. Cover your eyes and ears; put a blanket over your head; call your neighbor for help.

• Don't try changing your eating habits while you are becoming an Intrinsic Exerciser. Eating and weight loss or gain are so closely connected that you'll just confuse and frustrate yourself.

• Stop trying quick fixes that come in a bottle.

• Stop trying so hard. Exercise becomes fun once it's driven by a clear vision of your exercise self.

The whole idea of expunging the extrinsic is to free up your mind of the Outside-In clutter related to exercise. You want to be able to selectively attend to thoughts, feelings, and ideas that will begin to shape your possible exercise self.

Developing Your Physical Vision

While you are expunging the extrinsic, you can begin to establish a vision of yourself as an exerciser in two ways: exerimaging and a movement mission.

Exerimaging

Quick, what do you think about in those moments of waiting during the day? For example, you are standing in line at the grocery waiting for the world's slowest checker. What do you see? A slow checker. Nah! I see a guy dressed in blue tights, a long-sleeve shirt, and running shoes. He's running laps around a track to see how fast he can go. It's sunny but cool. He feels the cool air enter his lungs. He feels the power in his stride. He's gliding along like an otter sliding down a mud bank. What fun!

It's me.

That's me I see.

I see myself running tremendously.

Regular exercisers do these exerimaging exercises frequently. A study by Kimberly Gammage and her colleagues at the University of Western Ontario showed that both male and female regular exercisers used various kinds of mental images more often than low-frequency exercisers. This is exercise behavior change from the inside out. The idea is to begin to connect yourself to the exercise experience, to activate your vision. Exerimaging helps you develop a powerful vision. There are all kinds of ways to see yourself exercising, even when you aren't. Athletes use mental imagery all the time. Jack Nicklaus, Tiger Woods, Bill Russell, Michael Jordan, and Chris Evert are just a few of the elite performers who have practiced their sport in their mind. They have all used imagery to help them perform better, to be prepared, and to energize themselves. Exerimaging can do the same thing for you, only you'll be using it simply to help you become a regular exerciser. And there are countless opportunities to exerimage throughout the day in one minute or less.

The One-Minute Exerimage

Remember, the main point with exerimaging is that you are building a clear and strong exercise self, a physical vision of yourself exercising at some point in the future. In a sense, "you fake it till you make it." You keep working on images of yourself as an exerciser until it becomes a part of who you are. Here are some examples of when and how you can exerimage in one minute or less:

Shower. Taking a shower is such a mindless habit that your mind can certainly focus on other things. When I'm taking my morning shower, I visualize when, where, and how I'm going to exercise that day. You can visualize your entire day and where exercise fits in the picture. You see yourself exercising as a regular part of your day. If you're not planning to exercise that day, you see yourself moving a lot. You see yourself taking a 5-minute walk break — anything to get moving.

The Waiting Game. You can also develop your exercise self anywhere you have a few minutes of down time:

- Waiting for the bank teller at the drive-through window.

- Watching the kids at a youth sport practice.

- Sitting in a boring meeting.

- Waiting for a meeting with your boss.

- Riding the elevator to your penthouse headquarters.

- Listening to your friend go on and on about her "great weekend."

Sleep. Just before heading off to dreamland, you can see yourself exercising the next day. This may be the best time of the day to exerimage. Heather Hausenblas and her colleagues at the University of Western Ontario conducted a study that showed that 75 percent of regular exercisers practiced some form of mental imagery, and the largest percentage of them imagined themselves exercising most often before going to sleep.

You may think that all of this seems silly. But I'm telling you that regular exercisers are just having fun with their physical selves. The bottom line is to see yourself differently from what you are now, at least in terms of movement.

Your Movement Mission

Another strategy for activating your possible exercise self is to develop a movement mission statement. This statement is personal. Only you and your closest friends or family members should know about it. Once you develop it, keep it where you can see it or have quick access to it. Tape it to your computer, place it in your purse, keep it on your nightstand. The idea is to read it a few times each day, especially if you are just starting. Read it when you are struggling with your exercise — it will help you take action. Read it when your exercise is going well — it will help you celebrate your success.

These questions could guide your development of a movement mission statement:

- How do you like to feel?

- What are the feelings you like to have?

- Where does exercise fit in with those feelings?

- Can you get those feelings from exercise? How?

- What's the primary reason you want to exercise? Be careful with putting goals such as "I want to lose weight" on a mission statement. If you want to lose weight, ask yourself why. Is it to stay healthy? The mission statement must be written at this deeper level. How do you think exercise will connect with your life? Can it give you more energy so you can play with your grandchildren?

Here's my mission statement, which is on a Post-It attached to my computer and on a piece of paper in my wallet.

I like to exercise because it's one of the best activities I know to remind me of who I've been, who I am, and who I want to be. I've been an athlete all my life and my exercise helps me keep that connection; I'm a husband and father and exercise gives me the energy to live those roles to the

*best of my ability each day; and I want to be someone
who helps other people live their dream of an active lifestyle. By teaching myself about motivation and movement, I can teach others.*

Every time I read my movement mission, I get a new desire to move my body. And this takes just 30 seconds or
so. I read my movement mission when I'm feeling a little
burned out or when I need a little boost of motivation.

Your movement mission helps you create a strong and
clear physical vision, which can help you overcome many
mental barriers to exercise. The mission can remind you of
the kind of exerciser you want to be, which will give you
the resolve to push away any negative feelings. For instance, whenever you begin to feel embarrassed, which
makes you wonder if you should go to your aerobics class,
you can quickly squelch that feeling by reading your movement mission statement.

Take a few moments right now to write your movement
mission statement. Then you're ready for the next part of
vision.

The Specifics of Inner Vision

How do I want my exercise to make me feel? How does it
feel when I move my body? These questions relate directly
to developing an *inner vision* of exercise. This inner vision
is just as important for becoming an Intrinsic Exerciser as
the physical vision of the possible exercise self. If you don't
know how it feels when you move or how you want to feel
when you move your body, your exercise experience will be

more negative than positive, more work than inspiration. Then you'll come up with lots of reasons not to exercise because you won't enjoy it.

You probably aren't used to asking these questions connecting exercise and feeling. But this inner vision based on how you want to feel is crucial to performing any behavior over a long period of time. The notion of inner vision is based partly on the work of a colleague of mine, Doug Newburg, the director of performance education at the University of Virginia School of Medicine. I've been fortunate enough to work with Doug over the past few years to learn more about why *how you want to feel* is so important whenever you undertake any kind of performance. Here's what I've learned: being aware of how you want to feel in any activity makes it more likely that you will perform well and enjoy the activity, that is, make it a positive experience. It doesn't matter if it's performing surgery, playing an instrument, teaching a class, or exercising. The main idea here is to heighten your awareness of how you want your exercise to feel and then make it happen. Doug calls this "resonance" — when how you want to feel is matched up with the actual experience.

Resonance developed out of interviews with hundreds of outstanding performers from all walks of life — sports, business, music, and medicine. Doug interviewed these people over many years to find out how they live their lives and what it takes to be a top performer in the game of life. The secret Doug uncovered was that these folks loved themselves first, enjoying their lives long before they became great performers. All of them struggled through major setbacks and obstacles. The secret was how they lived before they were famous or successful. They knew how they wanted to feel every day, and then they went out and lived their life to achieve it. Great performers start with the question *"How do I want to feel each day?"* This is the driving inner force behind the lives of all great performers. Call it passion or magic. You are going to take this same idea and apply it to exercise. Knowing how you want to feel when you exercise and then making it happen is the best-kept secret in exercise behavior change.

I've been helping one exerciser work on identifying the feelings she wants to overcome—her feelings of intimidation—when she exercises around other people. Some of the feelings she has identified are "feeling useful and competent and the feeling of beauty and ritual." Whenever the negative feelings of intimidation or embarrassment begin to rise to the emotional surface, she replaces them quickly by reminding herself of the feelings she likes to have and how exercise helps her feel this way.

If you don't exercise now, you're probably wondering how you want to feel when you do exercise. But don't worry: the mind is powerful. All of us have had some positive feelings with movement, but many people have forgotten or suppressed them. You first need to develop an enhanced awareness of your own body and your own movement.

Enhanced body awareness leads to change. Many people are afraid to be self-aware because of what they think they might find out about themselves and their body. Ken Ravizza, a sports psychologist at California State University at Fullerton, writes, "Although it may be difficult to increase a person's awareness after he has neglected it for so long, a multitude of insights can be gained from daily occurrences, if one is willing to focus attention on bodily experiences."

This increased awareness will naturally lead to more frequent exercise. I can't help but use a nonexercise example to demonstrate the power of awareness.

My daughter used to have an Achilles' heel: she would pick and pull at her fingernails. Her nails were downright ugly, not to mention painful. One night my wife lit into her, telling her to stop this seemingly nonsensical behavior. That didn't work, so I talked with her about the situation. I ended by asking her to do one thing: just start to observe *when* you have this behavior. She looked at me as if I had lost my mind. "You mean you don't want me to stop," she said. I reminded her each morning and night to play this awareness game over the next few days. Then one night she burst into our room and said she knew when she was acting out. She was so proud of herself. She went on to tell me that she was going to just stop doing the behavior now that she knew why she was doing it. That clicked with me. You just catch yourself, tell yourself NO, and then say something positive to yourself, such as, "I really like the way my nails are looking."

The point of this story, of course, is to demonstrate that my daughter couldn't change her behavior until she was more aware of when she was doing it. And she couldn't become more aware until I helped her take the pressure — and focus — off the desired outcome (Outside-In). My point: you won't exercise the way you want to, won't change your behavior, until you become more aware of how and what you feel when you move your body. And there are many ways to do this.

Observations, Not Judge and Jury

Start by making simple observations about your movement patterns; you can keep a journal or log if you want. The main point is to not judge your body or your lack of regular movement as bad. Tim Gallwey, who wrote the *Inner Game* books, calls this "nonjudgmental awareness" — to see what is happening rather than noticing how well or how badly it is happening. The goal of observations is to learn more about your body and movement patterns. You begin to make observations, not judgments, about yourself and your physical activity. You don't place a value on the behavior. You simply step outside yourself and observe things such as

- moments when you feel like moving but don't
- moments when you could move but don't
- moments when you do move
- how you feel when you see other people moving
- how you feel when you move
- the situations you are in when you move
- the thoughts and situations that prevent your moving.

For example, I have a vision of myself as a mover. On days that I don't do any structured exercise, I could be quite in-

active. But I make sure my off days involve more movement. For instance,

- I walk to class (about 5 minutes).

- One day my students took a quiz in class. When each one
  of my 50 students was done, I walked around and picked
  up the quiz. This forced me to walk continuously for
  about 5 minutes.

- I take a tea break and walk over to our food court to buy
  a cup of tea and walk back.

- I make sure I do something active with my kids.

These activities help reinforce my exercise self (physical
vision) and help me get that positive feeling of being active
(inner vision). It keeps my Intrinsic Exerciser active. I've
been able to develop these light to moderate physical activity days because I'm aware of and plan situations that will
make me move more.

Dare to Be Aware
Fits the Lifestyle Approach

As you become more aware of your movement through observations, you will begin to perform light to moderate
physical activity when opportunities arise. If you've been
struggling with a traditional, structured exercise program,
you may want to try the *lifestyle* approach to exercise. The
idea here is to accumulate or build physical activity into
your daily routine. You can still get the 30 minutes per day;
you just don't get it all at once, the way you do in a struc-

tured session. Research reviewed by a panel of experts in the *Journal of the American Medical Association* shows that a minimum of two and a half hours of moderate physical activity a week can improve your health. And it doesn't seem to matter how you get that time. John Jakicic and his colleagues found that previously sedentary, overweight women who performed short bouts (about 10 minutes) of multiple exercise sessions five days a week adhered to the program as well as the women who exercised continuously for 30 to 40 minutes (and both groups lost equal amounts of weight). Another study found that men who jogged in three separate 10-minute sessions daily became as fit as those who jogged for 30 minutes at a session. A study by Andrea Dunn and her colleagues from the Cooper Institute for Aerobics Research in Dallas found that the frequency of long-term exercise was the same whether people followed a lifestyle or structured exercise program. And the good news is a recent study by Panteleimon Ekkekakis and his colleagues at the University of Illinois, who found that even short walks of 10 minutes can lift one's mood. Your body wants to move and you feel better when it does.

Moving your body more during the day might ease your time pressure a little bit and give you the confidence that you can exercise. Then you can try the structured approach again.

For instance, if you're at the airport, walk to the gate instead of taking the horizontal escalators. Climb the stairs rather than taking the escalator or the elevator. At lunchtime, go to a nearby park and walk for 10 or 15 minutes.

You really can't lose. Take some time to begin observing

your body and develop an awareness of when it wants to move. Then act on those urges. At the very least, start fidgeting more. That's right, fidget. One study at the Mayo Clinic found that fidgeters burn hundreds of extra calories a day. Start tapping those fingers and feet.

An Awareness Story

The best story I've heard about effectively using an awareness strategy for moving more comes from Kristi Nadler, a graduate student at Miami University. She wrote about her experience trying to become a regular exerciser after finishing high school: "During my high school days, I was always active, participating in three varsity sports: volleyball, basketball, and softball. With this, we had a minimum of two hours of practice on all nongame days with the exception of Sunday. In addition, I usually lifted and engaged in weight training activities two or three times per week as well. These structured physical activities allowed me to be extremely active and I was in top physical shape.

"It was not until after high school that I began to find many obstacles in the way of exercise. After all of that sport structure was eliminated, a physical activity void developed in my life. The organization and social aspect of sport was gone, and I had a difficult time dealing with this. There was a new sense of freedom when I no longer had a sport that consumed my free time. Instead of forcing myself to engage in physical activity for at least a portion of the free time I had, I started to become more social outside of the athletic world. In addition, I began feeling a sense of loss in no longer having structure in my life, and so I did not want to engage in anything related to what I had done for so many years.

"One day I decided that I was not going to mope any longer, so I attempted to get myself back into a routine. At this point, I just could not make myself work out for a consistent length of time (usually less than a week). This went on for quite a while. The cycle began with a new idea for exercise that I would try for a short amount of time, and then I would decide that I no longer wanted to participate in that activity. This continued for about a year and a half to two years, and the total amount of physical activity that I actually did during this period of time was about 60 to 75 days per year. This was pathetic, especially since I engaged in physical activity about 275 to 300 days per year when in high school.

"Finally, after a long stretch of engaging in virtually no physical activity at all, I began to develop a lifestyle plan, and at first, this happened without my realization. I began to engage in short bouts of movement throughout the day, taking an extra lap around the mall, parking in the farthest spot at the grocery store, making two to three trips up and down the basement steps when I only needed one. Before I knew it, I began to feel better again, and I noticed some changes in my body and my energy level. After this started, I also began to take short walks throughout the day around the block, or between classes.

"This lifestyle approach to physical activity helped to pull me out of the rut I was in, and has been the motivating factor that has kept me going with exercise. Currently, I find myself adding more structured exercise from time to time, but it is the lifestyle activities that hold the foundation of my physical fitness."

Kristi is not so different from Mary, whom I introduced at the beginning of this chapter, but Kristi has rediscovered the joy of movement. She let go of her past ideas about exercise and created new ones. She held on to her vision as an exerciser but through heightened awareness realized that her old approach — lots of structure — wasn't feeling right. It wasn't working. By observing her patterns throughout the day, she was able to act quickly on opportunities to be physically active. She didn't judge if those activities were helping her become fit, she just moved. Remember Forrest Gump? He just ran. But you'll do this only if you nonjudgmentally observe the patterns of your body and your movement, where and when you can start to move. Don't judge, just move.

An excellent example of how awareness is essential for successful behavior change appears in Neale Donald Walsch's best-selling *Conversations with God.* God tells Walsch, "Now there's one way to change all that [a behavior]. You have to change your thought about it. . . . If you want to change a root thought, you have to ACT before you think." When it comes to exercise, many of us have deeply ingrained root thoughts that aren't positive and probably aren't even true. And they stop us from moving. We think too much and we think wrong. We think of all the reasons not to exercise, which blinds us to the joy of movement. We are so paralyzed by our excuses and debilitative thinking that we cannot move our body.

Today, when you think of exercise, be prepared and act quickly, move. The next time you'll have less negative thought and more action. As God tells Walsch, "It's important now, it's time now, to *change your mind* about some things." So ACT before you think, and before you know it, you'll be thinking like an exerciser.

The Purposeful Movement Incident

At this point, you probably realize that inner vision is about how you want to feel when you move. I love the feelings I get when I'm active with my kids. It's not so much the activity but just being around them that makes me feel so good. So I'm always looking for opportunities to be around them. Once you are aware of how you want to feel physically and the situations that give you those feelings, you'll go to extreme lengths to obtain those feelings. Here's one of my extreme exercise examples:

The other day I was working in my office when I just had this feeling of missing my family. Then I had a brainstorm: I would try to run a course at noon that would take me on a path that might give me a glimpse of my son, when he would be in a car going to a program. It wouldn't be the same feeling as playing with him, but still it would be something. I hoped I would be running on the road right at that time. I realized that this plan had a good chance of failure, but at least I was moving my body. The prospect of seeing him kept me going throughout the run. As I was running up a hill, I saw the car I was looking for. As I ran by, I saw my son's winter hat. That's all I saw of him — his red and blue elf hat — which was so cute that the emotion welled up inside me as I ran. That "accidental" incident made my day.

The story reflects my inner vision. You can develop or uncover your inner vision — how you want to feel with exercise — in other ways as well.

Ancient Replay

This inner vision technique came to me when my son and I were playing basketball with his mini-hoop in the garage. He was pretending to be Michael Jordan and "dunked" one. He then said he wanted to do an "ancient replay." Of course, he meant to say "instant replay," but after I stopped laughing, I realized that ancient replay is a great technique for all of us to activate our Intrinsic Exerciser. The idea is simple. Go back and recall the times you enjoyed moving your body. And don't tell me you can't remember any. We all have them. If you need help, go back and look at pictures from your childhood. At least one shows you doing something physical and will help you rekindle those positive feelings of moving your body. Another approach is to write about your positive physical activity experiences when you were younger. Disregard the negative stuff, such as being picked last in physical education class. You want to replay only the positive movement experiences. Write about those. For example, I once wrote about running my favorite course when I go back to visit my parents in my hometown. During this run, I relive some of my childhood memories. I wrote this ancient replay for myself but on a whim sent it to *Runner's World*, which published it. Here's an excerpt:

> As I run out toward the lake, I head toward my childhood home. My yearning is stronger now, and memories and visions pull me along at a faster clip.
>
> I climb the three hills that tell me I'm getting closer. I spot the worn path that winds through the woods and out to the shore. We used to take our black Lab there and watch him leap into the water to fetch sticks. Go, Blackie!
>
> When I run around the bend in the path, the lake comes into full view. Its beautiful stillness reminds me of the freedom of my childhood, the only time I was truly home. The glimmering lake reflects memories of fishing, swimming, and pleasant, cool evenings with my family. I wonder if other families still come here today.
>
> Nearing my turnaround point, I see the remnants of the old Glenmere Hotel and its nine-hole golf course. By the time I was old enough to play golf, the course already was in disrepair. But Dad still taught me to play. I once shot a bird straight out of the sky with one of my errant drives. As I run through the woods, I feel the presence of the great Babe Ruth, who often came to the Glenmere with his hunting cronies back in the glory days.
>
> I turn around reluctantly and head back toward town. The lake is behind me now, as is my childhood. My home run will soon end, but once again it has served me well. I finish with a clearer understanding of where I've been, who I am, and what I want to become.

An entire science of reminiscence has been developed and is sometimes used as a form of therapy. You can use your own reminiscences to recall your favorite physical activities, especially focusing on the feelings you had when participating. You can focus your recall on questions such as:

Did you have a favorite physical activity as a child?

How did it make you feel?

Are there ways you can move your body now that would give you similar feelings?

What positive images and feelings of your physical life can you bring to life right now?

The sports psychologist Terry Orlick recommends a technique called *feelization*. He writes, "The most powerful imagery for nurturing positive connections between mind and body, body and mind, or one mind and another involves positive feelings. Thus, I call it feelization rather than visualization: it centers on feeling."

Use any technique that feels comfortable to you to evoke the positive feelings you once had about physical movement. The positive feelings are part of your inner vision. Once you access these feelings, you can use them to help you move more frequently. Don't let go of them. Don't forget them. As Paul Wong, an expert on aging and memory at Trinity Western University in Langley, British Columbia, writes, "It is through looking back that we learn what we have always wanted to do." The clues for your Intrinsic Exerciser now and in the future can be found in the positive feelings you once had toward physical activity and movement. I even go so far as to keep the exercise segment of *Forrest Gump* cued up. I then watch the clip when I'm sick or haven't been able to exercise in a while. Watching the tape always inspires me to go back to why I exercise: feelings of freedom, reflective opportunities, flow, or because

I just feel like running. It's very powerful, for watching the video evokes the memories and feelings of why I exercise.

The vision strategies in this chapter can help pull you through the times when you are deciding whether to go to yoga class, take a walk, ride your bike, or pump some iron. Evoking your positive images and feelings will help you decide to exercise rather than staying home or doing nothing. That's exercising from the inside out. Here's a summary of how to create your vision:

Physical Vision — The exerciser I know is possible

1. *Expunge the Extrinsic.* Avoid any information or products that are primarily Outside-In or extrinsic-oriented.

2. *Exerimage.* Use one-minute exerimage opportunities as often as possible. Visualize the kind of exerciser you want to be. What kind of exercise self do you want to be?

3. *Create your own Movement Mission.* Write down why you want to exercise and what the driving force is for you to move your body on a regular basis.

Inner Vision — How I want my exercise to feel

1. *Dare to be self-aware.* Start observing your movement patterns. Keep an activity journal if that helps increase your observations. Be as nonjudgmental as possible as this enhances awareness, which leads to change.

2. *Practice ancient replay.* Go back to your past physical activity and recall the positive movement experiences. Write them down. Tell them to your best friend. Recall

your favorite physical activities when younger and explore what it felt like when you moved your body.

3. *Go back to your future.* Connect your past movement experiences to how you want your exercise to feel now and in the future.

4. *Use media memories.* Find your favorite pieces from movies, songs, and poems that help you generate or recreate the positive feelings you associate with exercise.

5

....

Step 2: Stay on Track
with Mastery

> Our current society works in many ways to
> lead us astray, but the path of mastery is
> always there, waiting for us.
>
> — George Leonard, *Mastery*

You're developing a vision of yourself as an exerciser, and you've been observing and tinkering with how you want to feel when you move. These are good first steps. On this inner path, *mastery* is the second step in changing your behavior from the inside out. One aspect of becoming an Intrinsic Exerciser is to become hooked on the mastery of moving your body. The essence of mastery is that you base success on your own criteria, on your own terms. This definitely requires an Inside-Out focus on your part.

The Science of Mastery

According to motivational theorists in education, sport, and exercise psychology, people typically view achievement and success in two ways: ego focus and mastery focus. These two views guide our behavior and our experiences in very different ways.

People who primarily emphasize an ego focus are continually comparing themselves with other people based on ability (the Outside-In approach). These people define success as doing better than other people. They are constantly judging, measuring, and evaluating themselves against standards outside themselves, so they are always looking for tasks that will help them achieve that success with minimal effort. For example, in sports, these ego folks would rather win against an easy opponent than lose against a challenging one. An ego focus leads to questions such as "How can I do better than this other person?" "Should I avoid this situation because I'm not good enough?" "Did I win?" Avoid such people like the plague. Fortunately, they're pretty easy to identify — they're always talking about themselves.

A mastery focus is quite different. People who focus on mastery view success as working hard, developing new skills, learning, and improving. Such people use their own criteria for determining their success, not other people's achievements. They may compare themselves to others, but those comparisons do not determine their feelings of success. With a mastery focus, people ask questions such as "How can I best acquire this skill or master this task?"

"Should I try this activity to see what I might learn?" "How hard did I try?" Mastery people can always teach us and are a lot of fun to be around.

In my experience, many people who start exercise approach it with an ego focus. But the research clearly shows that virtually always approaching exercise with a mastery focus is far better.

Mastery Leads to Perceived Competence

People with low ability perceive greater ability when they emphasize a mastery focus. A mastery focus keeps you in tune with your own ability and improvement. So when you start to improve, you'll notice it and you'll feel great.

A few years ago, preparing for a workshop on physical activity and older adults, I interviewed a YMCA member. He was a businessman in his seventies but, more important, ran marathons and played volleyball. He didn't start exercising until his forty-seventh year. When I asked him how he did it, he said something along the lines of "one step at a time." He started by walking around outside his YMCA. Then he started walking around the block. Then he walked 1 mile out and 1 mile back. Then he jogged the 2 miles. Then he jogged farther. Then he started running. Then he ran farther. After he described this amazing sequence of improvement, I asked him what had kept him going through the months when most people would have quit early on. His answer: "I got great pleasure out of seeing what I could do next. I loved improving." He didn't compare himself with others. He exercised to the beat of his own mastery drum. It is the best way. Zoom in on your performance and you'll find that you'll be much happier, a better performer — and an Intrinsic Exerciser.

Mastery Helps with Effort and Persistence and Builds Confidence

People with a mastery focus try harder and persist longer than those with an ego focus. Effort and persistence are crucial for exercising on a regular basis. If you have an ego focus, you may get discouraged quickly because you will always be comparing yourself to other people. If you're inexperienced, you can't possibly match up. One of my former research mentors, Joan Duda, now at the University of Birmingham in England, did a study a number of years ago showing that people who emphasized mastery, or what she calls "task involvement," responded to the exercise experience in a much more positive way than individuals who emphasized how their exercise performance compared to that of other ego-oriented people. The mastery folks responded to exercise with more of a "feel good" response. The same amount of physical work was perceived as less fatiguing. Don't you think you'll persist with exercise longer if it feels good and is less fatiguing?

If you enter an exercise program with an ego focus, you are in for a bumpy ride. One of the bumps is physique anxiety — the uneasy feeling you have when you compare your body with those of others. Face it: our society suggests that your body should look a certain way, so when you get into certain situations where your body may be judged by others

— swimming pools, health clubs — you can experience physique anxiety if you don't think your body measures up.

Don't underestimate the power of behavioral paralysis that physique anxiety or feelings of embarrassment hold over you. A survey of 1,180 sedentary adults conducted by America Sports Data showed that 37 percent of those who considered themselves overweight said they would be more receptive to joining a health club if they were less intimidated by the members. In addition, 46 percent of those overweight felt a need for a special program for out-of-shape beginners; 23 percent wanted to exercise in a private room away from the "hardbodies."

If you carry an ego focus into these physically toxic situations, you are really in trouble. You can't help but be self-conscious and nervous because your body and performance will not likely compare well with those of the more experienced exercisers.

I know both male and female faculty and staff at Miami University who will not set foot in our beautiful Recreation Center because they are inhibited by the 18- to 21-year-old bodies working out beside them. Women in particular face this issue. A study by Linda Bain at California State University–Northridge and her colleagues found that the most powerful barrier to exercise participation for overweight women was their concern about visibility and being judged, both by the instructors and by other members of the facility. Women are almost forced to compare their bodies with society's extreme, unattainable standards of low weight and beauty.

Step 2: Stay on Track with Mastery

One thing I've learned from talking with women who have become exercisers and lost weight in the process is that they stopped comparing themselves with other women or an unattainable standard and zoomed in on the behavior and experience itself. They either found environments that allowed them to let go or they decided that they didn't care what people thought of their bodies. They then became better at the physical activities they were trying to do and found that mastery makes exercising quite enjoyable and — voilà! — they lost weight naturally after a while.

Numerous studies have shown that individuals high in confidence, which is partly influenced by mastery experiences, are more motivated to exercise than individuals who are not confident — they work harder and persist longer. For instance, a study by one of the leaders in exercise adherence research, Edward McAuley, and his associates at the University of Illinois showed that confident exercisers are more intrinsically motivated to exercise. If you develop a strong sense of success based on your own criterion (mastery), in the process you will gain more confidence in your physical abilities and gradually, inevitably, transform yourself into an Intrinsic Exerciser. Is that a good enough reason to uncover the magic of mastery? Rita Callahan did.

Rita Callahan, at 47, was overweight and out of shape. A small business owner and mother of three in San Diego, she didn't like it that she was having a hard time walking upstairs. She couldn't keep up with her children. She had tried exercising and losing weight many times in the past with no success. Then a fitness coach helped her to begin focusing on mastery. "Don't worry about what other folks are doing," she said. "Concentrate on your own goals and what you are capable of doing." She had a simple approach: "Just come and get dressed. Sign in. Do the smallest thing. Just get yourself used to coming in and getting on the treadmill. It doesn't matter how much you accomplish right at first. We'll build up. We'll do a little bit at a time."

Rita was smart enough to realize that mastery was the way to go with her exercise. "I don't know when it really turned around," she says. "But it wasn't very long before I realized, number one, I can do this, and number two, I can actually make progress, because that was a big thing. I tried not to worry that other people were running or walking 25, 30, or 40 minutes. I was happy when I walked 1 minute longer than the time before." Rita kept progressing until she was exercising 4 or 5 days a week. (By the way, Rita eventually lost 78 pounds. The wizardry of weight loss lies in the magic of exercise mastery.)

Rita was lucky: she was able to exercise in an area that was separate from the general exercise area, which helped her deemphasize comparisons with other people. But even if this isn't the case for you, the same approach will help you.

One of the best ways to build a sense of mastery and confidence is through pictures and videotapes of you or others like you performing the desired behavior. Stacy Wegley, a health educator with the Hamilton County General Health District in Cincinnati, has used this strategy successfully with her clients. She started up a chair volleyball league for older women but was having some difficulty getting them to play because they didn't think they could do it. "Many older adults, especially women, have no experience with physical activity and they have the perception that they are unable to be physically active, especially in a game setting," says Wegley. She initially tried to have them think about joining in by having them talk themselves into it, but she found what worked best was to have the better players demonstrate the game for those who were tentative. She now shows a video of players and action pictures to newcomers. "I can see the newcomers' faces light up when they see other people even older than they are playing the game," says Wegley. "They just get more confident and say, 'If they can do it, so can I.' Hazel Ellis, at 80, was reluctant at first but now says, "I put my all into chair volleyball, I love it so much. It gets you out with your friends. It's a lot of exercise. I hope I play for 10 more years."

Also, using a step-by-step mastery approach can boost your confidence. Tony Poggiali, the former fitness director at Maple Knoll Wellness Center in Cincinnati, would conduct three progressive, personal run-throughs with every new member. Many of these people were at least 70 years old, and, as all of us are at first, they were uncertain how to proceed with strength machines. Tony's goal was "to take each member to a state of confident independence." The first time, he did most of the talking and some demonstration. On the second visit, he guided the member through the equipment and answered any questions. And on the third one, he told the member to act as if he were not there.

"I would usually see a big change from the first to third run-through," says Poggiali. "Many of the members went from timidly walking in there to walking in with a swagger and an 'I know what I'm doing' attitude. Without the three run-throughs, I don't think anyone would have shown up."

You can do what Tony did with his clients. Break down your exercise into manageable tasks and progress. Each mini-success along the way builds your confidence.

Mastery Makes You a Quality Performer

People with a mastery focus choose tasks of appropriate difficulty, whereas those with an ego focus typically choose tasks that are too hard or too easy. Because people with a mastery focus are interested in learning, developing skills, and improving, they pick exercise tasks that are challenging but realistic. They naturally select activities matched with their ability.

Face it: most of us want to perform well when we exercise — or when we do anything, for that matter. Quality performances make us feel good about ourselves. Having a mastery focus is the best way to make your exercise a quality experience each time. Terry Orlick writes, "I have never encountered an athlete who had an all-time best performance while focusing on winning or losing during an event. The problem with thinking about winning or losing within an event is that you lose focus of what you need to do in order to win."

Mastery guides you to quality exercise experiences, which will also motivate you to exercise more frequently.

My colleagues and I conducted a study in which the results showed that high mastery–oriented members of an exercise program exercised more frequently and were likelier to achieve their goals than low mastery–oriented members. A mastery focus helps you enjoy your exercise more because you'll be successful more often and it makes you a better performer.

Susan Jackson, an optimal experience researcher formerly at the Queensland University of Technology in Queensland, Australia, interviewed a group of masters athletes at all levels of ability and found that mastery was central not only to why they enjoy exercise but also to why they continue to exercise. Reading through the interview transcripts, she and I found that comments relating to mastery far exceeded comments relating to ego reasons for exercising.

Here's what one male swimmer in his early fifties had to say relating to mastery:

> You are not worrying about what other people think. If you were worried about that you won't be here racing. In Masters it doesn't matter how good or bad your are, you just have a go and you only go against yourself, that's what it's all about. If you win, you win. If you don't win a trophy, you are still a winner. . . . My main goal is to try and break my own time and to do my best.

And here's a mastery quote from a 49-year-old female triathlete:

> It's against myself that's most important. I just set my own sort of goals. I know I'm a realist, so I know where I am in

89

terms of my physical fitness. I don't really worry about everybody else. I just worry about myself and see how I sort of manage to get through it.

The effects of mastery on experience start at a young age. For a number of years, I've been interested in the effect that mastery has on children's physical activity patterns. With my colleague Thelma Horn, I have published a series of studies that demonstrate that kids with a high mastery orientation for exercise and physical fitness are more physically active than kids that are low in mastery. And do you know what is one of the most significant factors that affect the degree to which kids emphasize mastery? It's to what extent the parents emphasize mastery for their children. Parents who help their kids focus on their own improvement, their own goals for physical activity, are more likely to activate a mastery focus in their children than parents who do not emphasize mastery.

Take a minute to determine if you now have more of a mastery or ego focus in terms of exercise. Again, be honest. You are only doing this for yourself.

YOUR EXERCISE FOCUS

Place a check next to all the statements that apply to you. Mark only those that would make you feel very successful. I would consider myself most successful with my exercise when

❑ 1. I lost a lot of weight as a result of exercising.

❑ 2. I learned something new about my body.

❑ 3. I could lift more weights than my friends.

❏ 4. I gave out a lot of effort during my exercise.

❏ 5. I was the best in my exercise class.

❏ 6. I did something with my exercise that I couldn't do the last time.

❏ 7. My body looked better than those of most people my age.

❏ 8. I learned to do a new exercise activity.

Scoring:
Add up your checks for numbers 1, 3, 5, and 7 _____ Ego total
Add up your checks for numbers 2, 4, 6, 8 _____ Mastery total

---

Ideally, you would like to have as many checks for mastery as ego. This means you are on the right track for developing a mastery focus. If your ego total outnumbered the mastery total, you have some mastery work to do. The mastery strategies outlined next should help.

Setting Goals and Changing Exercise Behavior

You need to tread lightly when setting behavioral goals, such as deciding to exercise 3 days a week for 6 weeks. Exercise adherence research shows us that setting goals that are too rigid can backfire and sabotage our motivation. If you miss your goal the first week, you may start thinking that you will stop exercising altogether. The study on overweight women in Chapter 4 suggested that women with minimal experience with behavior change are very susceptible to this kind of demotivating thought process.

Being flexible with your goals is much better. One

woman in the overweight women study "noted that when she gave herself permission not to exercise or to exercise according to her mood, it was easier to view exercise as a choice and to maintain her subsequent participation." A study by John Martin and his associates at the Veterans Administration Medical Center in Jackson, Mississippi, found that flexible goals led to greater exercise adherence than goals that were fixed and rigid.

Before we continue, you have to make the following promise: Over the next 6 months, perhaps forever, I will not set any weight loss goals, weigh myself, or compare my body or my progress with that of other people. Also, I will not motivate myself to exercise because of promised rewards.

Work on the mastery component of the Intrinsic Exerciser, make a commitment to uncovering the kind of mover you were meant to be, and set only those goals that internalize your motivation. Instead of focusing on outcomes, goals can focus on process or experience. Exercise goals that connect to your natural inner needs for movement are the most effective for behavior change.

Remember, mastery implies that you base your success on your own criteria. Any exercise goal should be yours and yours alone, and you are the one who determines the degree of achievement. Use the power of setting goals to focus your mind and body on learning, improving, feeling, and experiencing. Your mind and body want to do these things naturally. Mastery puts you in charge.

Part of the fun is figuring out which mastery goal you are going to set for any given day of exercise. The only rule is that you set at least one goal for every exercise session. The goal gives your mind an intrinsic focus for that particular movement experience (your mind needs something to focus on to optimize the experience). Before you start, you should write down your mastery goal. After a while, you'll be able to state your mastery goal according to how you feel that day. In this section, I'll show you how to set the following four mastery goals: *Learning*, *Improvement*, *Feeling*, and *Experiencing*. This L.I.F.E. approach will work for the rest of your life.

Learning Goals

The intent of *learning goals* is to maximize your inner desire to learn through moving your body. Ask yourself questions such as, What do I want to learn today through exercise? Do I want to learn to concentrate better? Do I want to learn about other people? Do I want to learn more about myself? Learning goals, as with all mastery goals, are designed to interest you while you are moving your body.

For example, I was at my parents' house with the kids during a spring break. On a day I chose to run outside, it started pouring as I was changing into my running gear. My initial goal was to try to improve my time on a course that I had run two days earlier. However, I was a little tired and the rain wasn't helping my motivation. I spotted my mother's treadmill in the corner and figured, what the heck, I'll try the treadmill. I asked my mom to show me how it works. I think she was quite proud that she could explain something to her son about exercise. My goal simply became to learn something about myself and my body while on the treadmill. I had a great time for 35 minutes, piddling around with the speed and the incline gadgets. I learned that treadmills aren't as boring as I had thought, that my knee didn't hurt as much as when I run outdoors on pavement. You get the idea. My simple learning goal enabled me to enjoy my treadmill exercise experience.

What kinds of learning goals can you set for your exercise? What do you want to learn about your body? About yourself? You can put your goals into several categories.

With *improvement goals*, you challenge yourself to get better or to do more. Your goal can be to walk 1 more minute than the time before or lift 2.5 pounds more on each piece of resistance equipment. Or you can do 1 more rep. Improvement can also be mental. You can have a goal to get better at something, such as concentrating while exercising. You can set a goal of maximizing stress reduction so that you are at peace before, during, and after a workout. Improvement implies accomplishment, but it does not have to be earth-shattering. As long as you improve, rejoice in that. The beauty is that you pick your goals based on where you are now. Set the intrinsic goal relevant to you so that it will pack a real punch for you.

Feeling goals help build the inner vision you want when you exercise. Such a goal may be to experience strength or speed. With cycling, sometimes you can try going fast; other times you can cycle slowly and really tune in to your legs' pumping. You may feel the need to be social, which could be attained by walking at noontime with colleagues at work or in the morning or evening with friends. You need to have a notion about how you want your movement to feel so that you can target your physical activity on that feeling. It may not be the same feeling every single time you exercise. The *YPersonal Fitness Program*, the 12-week exercise behavior change program that I helped develop with the YMCA of the USA, has a goal-setting component in line with the feeling goal. Members decide if they want to feel better, energized, or confident, for example. Then they focus on ways to move their body to help them get that feeling.

And there are *experience goals*, which focus on your senses — at least sight, touch, hearing, and smell. My goal is often to experience my senses, one at a time, throughout my workout. If I'm in a strange location or a little burned out on exercise, this goal always leaves me refreshed. I try to see something new in my environment; I focus on my feet striking the pavement; I guess at the sounds and smells around me, where they are coming from and if they are pleasant. By focusing on your senses, you not only maximize the experience but have a different experience than you may have had before. Because I set different mastery goals all the time, my experience with exercise always differs.

6

....

Step 3: Stay in the Moment
with Flow

> Flow is a source of psychic energy in that it
> focuses attention and motivates action.
>
> — Mihaly Csikszentmihalyi, *Finding Flow*

Once, when I was to give the closing address at a conference held in a park, I was looking forward to a pleasant evening and half a day there. But when I arrived, the weather
was absolutely terrible — rain, fog, and cold. It was so bad
that I put off a run until the next morning. But that plan
proved no better. I got into my running clothes through
pure habit and stumbled outside. At 6:30 A.M., the sky was
pitch-black, so I couldn't see anything. For some reason, I
felt drawn to the darkness. I pushed my hat down low and
ventured slowly into the black. My biggest fear was trip-
ping and hurting myself. I almost turned back — and then

my eyes caught sight of the white line, the line that indicates where road and shoulder meet.

The line became my mantra during the entire run, guiding my way. Although my initial plan was to run 15 minutes out and the same amount back, I became so wrapped up with the run that I didn't check my watch the way I typically do. I remembered only after 20 minutes.

On the way back, I thought about the only other time in my life that I remembered the white line being so important. In seventh grade I went to a meeting with my father, and on the drive home we hit dense fog. My dad told me to help him by keeping my eye on the white line. I was scared, but I also felt important. We made it through the fog and arrived home safely.

After my run, a peace came over me along with a boost of energy that carried me through my address. What I experienced that day was what is commonly called "flow." Nothing was extraordinary about the experience, but it was pleasant because I stayed in the moment and felt revived later. You need this experience. Exercise without flow is like sex without love or New Year's Eve without champagne. Often you can create and construct an exercise experience to make flow more likely.

Here is how two regular exercisers describe their flow experiences:

> It's like real high energy. I'm feeling good, feeling in control, feeling like I don't want it to stop. I'm not concerned at all with what's around me. I'm just focused on what's going on in my head.

I love activity. I think I just love the feeling you get from it. I know that I love watching a person playing a sport, just to see the energy that goes into it.

Flow, which is a hot topic in the sport and exercise psychology literature, is a positive psychological state that occurs when a person is intently absorbed in an activity. The idea is simple and helps you enjoy your involvement so much that you want to do it repeatedly. You will even go to great lengths to do so. For instance, I always take my running clothes on trips because I become interested in new surroundings, and enter flow easily then. Csikszentmihalyi has described several characteristics of flow during his years of research: challenge-skill balance, the merging of action and awareness, clear goals and feedback, total concentration on the task at hand, a sense of control, a loss of self-consciousness, time transformation, and an intrinsically rewarding experience. You should be attuned to these dimensions so that you can get better at developing the flow mentality in your physical activity experiences.

For instance, you have a good chance of experiencing flow when you perceive that the challenges of the situation and your skills are in balance. If there is an imbalance, it is highly unlikely that you will experience flow. More likely you will experience anxiety or boredom. Anxiety occurs when you perceive the challenges of the situation to be higher than your perceived skills; boredom results when your skills outweigh the challenges. Typically, the quality of your exercise experience will be best in flow, worst when you experience boredom or anxiety.

Step 3: Stay in the Moment with Flow

Flow in Exercise: A Balance Between Challenge and Skill

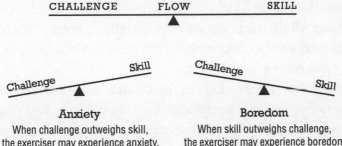

Anxiety	Boredom
When challenge outweighs skill, the exerciser may experience anxiety, leading to dropout or sporadic physical activity.	When skill outweighs challenge, the exerciser may experience boredom and frustration, leading to dropout or infrequent physical activity.

Second, the merging of action and awareness suggests that your involvement in an activity is so deep that it becomes spontaneous or automatic. Simply, you become one with the activity. Susan Jackson, a research colleague, has found that many elite athletes describe this flow dimension as "being in the groove" or "I am not thinking about anything . . . it just happens automatically."

And the characteristics of clear goals and feedback go together like exercise and sweat. To get into flow, your goals must be clearly defined by either planning ahead or developing them while engaging in the activity. When you know and understand the goals, it is more likely that you will become totally immersed or engaged. What's more, a clear goal makes processing feedback easier, which provides messages that you are progressing with the goal. The powerful link between goals and feedback creates a mental harmony, which is at the core of the flow experience. The mastery goals outlined earlier are actually a means of getting you into flow.

Total concentration is also important. The complete focus on the task at hand stands out as the clearest indication of flow. All distractions are nonexistent or kept at a minimum, and only a select range of information is allowed into your awareness.

Moreover, when you are in flow, you feel in control of the situation and don't worry about losing control. You must have a sense of what Csikszentmihalyi calls "exercising control in difficult situations." For instance, when it's a bit crowded in the weight room, can you block out any distractions and control your mental processes enough to have an enjoyable session?

When you're in flow, no room exists for distractions or worry about how you are perceived by others. Because self-consciousness does not enter in, a sense of separateness from the world is overcome. The result is a feeling of oneness with the environment. The absence of self-consciousness does not mean that you are not aware of your thoughts and bodily movements. Rather, it is a keen awareness that is not threatening. In essence, your self is fully functioning but not aware of doing it.

The perception of time may also speed up or slow down in flow, for time is distorted by the experience. For example, you get so into an aerobics class that it seems as if it ended more quickly than it actually did. You know you are in flow when 30 minutes on the stair-stepper seems to be only a few minutes. Flow transcends time. This happened to me with my "white line" flow experience.

The result of flow is intrinsically rewarding. Statements such as "I really had a great experience" illustrate the product of a flow experience. A flow state is so positive that you begin to want to perform the activity for its own sake.

Getting in the Exercise Groove

Are you a flowmeister? Think about your typical physical experiences and how often you get into flow. Never? Some of the time? All the time? The goal is not that you'll experience flow every single time you exercise but that you will develop a mental and emotional approach to exercise that makes it more likely that you can sometimes "get in the groove." This will make your exercise more enjoyable. Here are some questions to help you understand your experience of flow during exercise:

- Do I frequently experience a balance between my physical skills and the physical challenge when I exercise?

- Do I sometimes feel as if I'm on automatic pilot, or am I spontaneous when I exercise?

- Do my mind and body feel connected at least some of the time when I exercise?

- Do I usually exercise without worrying about what others might be thinking of me?

- Does time sometimes go by quickly, or does 20 minutes seem like an eternity when I move my body?

- At least some of the time, do I have an inner glow after movement?

If you answered yes to most of these questions, you are a flowmeister in exercise; you enjoy your exercise often because of flow experiences. If you answered no to a few of these questions, fear not. You can teach yourself the mental skills needed to get into flow more frequently.

Much overlap exists between mastery and flow. Mastery prepares you for flowlike exercise experiences. And without flow, you will find all kinds of excuses not to work out. You can connect mastery and flow in almost any physical activity. For example, setting a clear mastery goal for your aerobics class helps you focus on the goal and process the feedback pertaining to the goal during the class. Mastery goals help you tune out irrelevant feedback or distractions so you can zoom in during your walk. These seem like simple tasks, but they work wonders for enhancing your exercise experiences. The mastery-flow connection comes directly from theory and research in sport and exercise psychology. A study by Susan Jackson and Glyn Roberts, now at the Norwegian University of Sport and Physical Education in Oslo, found that athletes high in mastery experienced flow more frequently than athletes low in mastery. Moreover, it found that athletes were primarily mastery-focused when describing best performances and more ego-focused when describing worst performances. The scientists also found that flow was experienced more in best performances than in worst performances.

In other words, mastery focuses you on the task at hand and flow enables you to have a quality experience, which then allows you to perform to the best of your ability. People of all ages and abilities can and do experience flow, especially when they are physically active. Research by Csikszentmihalyi and his colleagues showed that teenagers were in flow 44 percent of the time when participating in games and sport, which was more than experienced in any other teenage activities. If teens can make it happen, so can you.

Beyond Exercise Performance

I've talked about flow making you a better performer while you exercise, but it does much more.

Flow generates positive emotions. For instance, a study with elite figure skaters found that a source of positive emotions for them was their sense of flow during skating. Children's flow experiences at a summer sports camp were related to "feeling good" and "perceived success."

Flow puts you in control. When you're in flow, external circumstances do not determine your experience. You'll enjoy yourself whatever the conditions, such as bad weather or too many people around you, because controlling your inner experience is easier than controlling your external environment.

Flow builds your concentration and attention. You become more aware of the mind-body connection. As you improve your concentration during exercise, the outcomes become less important. Csikszentmihalyi writes, "The important thing is to enjoy the activity for its own sake, and to know that what matters is not the result, but the control one is acquiring over one's attention."

With a little practice, you can teach yourself how to keep your mind in the present during exercise. David Brown and his colleagues conducted a study at the University of Massachusetts Medical School in Worcester that taught people to repeat the word "left" or "right" every time the appropriate foot struck the ground during a walk. The goal was to stay with this mantra as long as possible during each exercise session. I've tried a variation of this, but first found I could only do it for a few minutes before other thoughts entered my mind. With practice, I've been able to increase my mantra time to about 10–15 minutes. It's an awesome experience.

Reaching a Plateau

After a while, low-impact aerobics or a slow walk around the block may not seem interesting to you. This is where mastery goals come into play. Set improvement goals for yourself — raise the stakes. Go to a higher-impact aerobics class or take faster walks around the block. Raise the challenge in some way, shape, or form.

Many people who focus on losing weight via exercise usually stumble at this point. They get bored and quit. Losing weight is hard work, and it's even harder if you're not having any fun doing it. The National Weight Control Registry shows that for people successful at losing at least 30 pounds and keeping the weight off for at least one year, exercising regularly was the key to their success. To be eligible for the registry, a person must have lost at least 30 pounds and maintained it for at least a year. Many of the members are very successful, having lost an average of 66 pounds and kept it off for an average of six years. Most of these people reported burning about 400 calories a day through walking, which was the most popular exercise. That's a lot of walking — about 60 to 90 minutes a day. I doubt if these folks would walk that much if they weren't finding ways to enjoy the experience at least some of the time.

Joann Donnelly, the metro director of health and fitness for the YMCA of Memphis, uses this up-the-challenge strategy to help her members work past plateaus in their exercise program. Donnelly uses treadmill training for the women. She helps them gradually raise their speed and has them gauge their physical sensations as the intensity increases. "Women love treadmill training," says Donnelly. "It puts them in touch with their feelings of exertion, and it really surprises them to see what they can do with their body."

You don't have to use a treadmill to get you over the boredom hump. It can be anything that makes your exercise a tad more difficult or different so that you have to concentrate.

If all else fails, I give you permission to go out and buy an exercise toy. For instance, you can buy a step counter to see the number of steps you take in a day. Supposedly, 10,000 steps is a healthy number. I haven't tried this, but people tell me it's fun.

Be smart, though, when you begin to up the challenge. Don't challenge yourself too far beyond your skill because you may enter the anxiety zone, which you want to avoid. Also, you want to be in a safe physical zone so that you don't injure yourself.

Tune In to Your Own Feedback

When you are done exercising, ask yourself questions such as how your body feels and what you were thinking about. Consider if the answers relate to the goal you set for that specific workout.

To help people tune in to flow feedback, I offer a self-guided flow form. Complete the form immediately after exercising to enhance your awareness of your experience. Occasionally review your completed forms to stay in touch with which activities produce flow and which ones do not.

SELF-GUIDED FLOW FORM

Date/time of exercise session: _____
Date/time form filled out: _____

Briefly describe your exercise session:
Who were you with (if anyone)? _____
Did you have a goal(s) for this exercise session? ❏ Yes ❏ No
If Yes, describe the goal(s). _____

	not at all	somewhat	quite	very
How enjoyable was the activity?	0 1 2	3 4 5	6 7 8	9
Am I satisfied with how I did?	0 1 2	3 4 5	6 7 8	9
Did I attain my goal(s)?	0 1 2	3 4 5	6 7 8	9
How well was I concentrating?	0 1 2	3 4 5	6 7 8	9
Was I in control of the experience?	0 1 2	3 4 5	6 7 8	9
Did the activity challenge me?	0 1 2	3 4 5	6 7 8	9
Was my skill level a good match with the activity?	0 1 2	3 4 5	6 7 8	9

Step 3: Stay in the Moment with Flow

Circle the response that *best* describes how you were feeling *immediately following* this exercise session:

	very	quite	some	neither	some	quite	very	
happy	O	o	•	—	•	o	O	sad
alert	O	o	•	—	•	o	O	drowsy
proud	O	o	•	—	•	o	O	ashamed
excited	O	o	•	—	•	o	O	bored
relaxed	O	o	•	—	•	o	O	tense
strong	O	o	•	—	•	o	O	weak
cheerful	O	o	•	—	•	o	O	irritable
active	O	o	•	—	•	o	O	passive

My flow notes:

7

....

Step 4: Fuel the Physical Fire with Inergy

> The ultimate reality of the universe is neither matter nor spirit but wholes.
>
> — Jan Smuts, *Holism and Evolution*

Inergy connects your movement or exercise with your other life needs, mental, social, and spiritual, and is based on the science and philosophy of wellness. Just focusing on exercise in one dimension — the physical — has a minimal motivational effect on most people. It focuses on the physical benefits of exercise but ignores the potential integration of exercise with mental, social, and spiritual needs — what I call "extreme wellness." As an Intrinsic Exerciser, you move toward extreme wellness through Inergy.

Understanding Your Mental, Social, and Spiritual Needs

Consider your other three needs separately and how exercise can help them. Our mental need refers to our need to learn. The intrinsic motivation experts Deci and Ryan suggest that this need is an innate feature of being human. But the wellness literature shows that it is more than a basic desire to learn. It also pertains to a variety of other desires, such as expressing and recognizing our feelings, controlling stress, and solving problems. Our mental need can also refer to thinking creatively and learning new skills. As a function of being human, we all have basic psychological needs, and exercise can help you meet those needs. A number of exercise psychologists have studied the role of exercise in helping people meet their mental needs.

For example, Abby King and her colleagues at Stanford University took a group of previously sedentary, middle-aged adults and put them on an exercise program for 6 months. They examined changes in psychological well-being every 2 weeks in both the exercise group and a control group of nonexercisers. Their findings show that the exercising group experienced rapid positive changes in their satisfaction with their body shape and appearance, weight, and fitness. In other words, their perception of their body changed as a result of moving their body. And the most dramatic changes occurred in the first month of the program, before any major physical changes actually occurred. The exercising group started to feel better about their body in a short amount of time, which indicates a strong link between movement and mental well-being.

Is 2 to 4 weeks too long for you to wait for the mental and emotional benefit of exercise? Well, you don't have to. The study I described in Chapter 4 on the quick mood-enhancing effects of walking is relevant here. That research showed that a 10- to 15-minute leisurely outdoor walk was associated with greater feelings of pleasure and greater energy.

Both of these studies are good news for the Intrinsic Exerciser. You can experience tremendous mental boosts from moving your body before you ever lose weight or get fit. The psychologist Thomas Plante at Santa Clara University writes, "Positive psychological benefits associated with exercise occur in good part because of the value one attributes to the process of becoming fit rather than primarily to actual aerobic physical fitness . . . perception of fitness may be more closely associated with improvements in psychological functioning than is aerobic physical fitness."

A study by Robert Motl and his associates at the University of Wyoming found that the rock climbers who enjoyed their experience the most demonstrated the greatest change in mood after an expedition. That is, the ones who enjoyed it relieved greater amounts of tension, felt more vigorous, and were less depressed and confused after climbing than before. These positive feelings can last for some time following exercise. A study by Lise Gauvin, a researcher at the University of Montreal, and her colleagues showed that the positive mood-enhancing effects of exercise — such as feelings of tranquility, revitalization, and positive engagement — lasted throughout the day, hours after the exercise occurred. And here's the kicker: the worse you feel before exercise, the better you feel afterward. An awareness of only this fact tips the scales in favor of working out on those days when you really don't want to. And this enhanced awareness keeps you out of negative or bad moods. When people are in a bad mood, they end up thinking about how bad all of their problems are. But when they're in a positive mood, which they can get from exercise, they can reflect on their life and see it in a positive light. And they are more likely to address their problems in ways that can solve them. Many opportunities exist in the course of your day to make the connection between physical exercise and your mental need. For example, on your next walk you can mull over a serious problem. Or you can enter a 5K run or walk to see how you do and thus learn something new.

Next, consider our social needs, which relate to communication and interactions with other people. These include respecting yourself and others, interacting with people, appreciating their differences, and creating and maintaining relationships.

To be an Intrinsic Exerciser, although you need to feel connected to other people, you do not always have to exercise with someone else. But as John Bingham, a columnist for *Runner's World*, writes, "I know now that there are also days when it isn't the miles but the people who are the most important part of the training. There are times when

111

sharing the joy of running, with a single individual or group, is necessary to complete myself."

I get most of my social support for exercise from my family. My wife listens patiently to my description of my run. She allows me to run when she quietly wishes I would not. And my kids love coming to the track with me. For me, seeing them run around the track with abandon motivates me to keep going when I don't really feel like it.

For example, several months ago I was home alone with my children for about three days. First we went ice skating and probably fell more times than we skated around the rink. Then we went to a gymnastics room and had the whole place to ourselves. My daughter performed a floor routine so spontaneous and energized that it blew me away. My son and I tried to hula hoop. That inergistic time stayed with me for a long, long time.

Research repeatedly shows that social support is a crucial factor in our ability not only to exercise but to change other health behaviors, such as quitting smoking and altering eating habits. Individuals who perceive a high level of social support exercise more frequently than those who don't. What's more, strong evidence now exists that positive social support can reduce your risk of a variety of diseases or risk factors, such as high blood pressure and stress.

For at least 6 months, the women that make up the administrative staff in our department have been walking on the indoor track at noon most days of the week. They tell me it's the first time they've ever maintained exercise for any length of time. They support each other. They talk

Step 4: Fuel the Physical Fire with Inergy

while walking and motivate each other to head over to the track when one of them doesn't feel like going.

This social support process occurs no matter how young or old you are. McAuley and his associates examined the link between exercise, social relations, and life satisfaction of formerly sedentary adults between the ages of 60 and 75. They found that the social relations that developed among the exercisers was the critical factor in determining their satisfaction with life at a one-year follow-up.

Exercise is a great way to meet basic social needs. For instance, if you are lonely or bored, you can join a walking group, an orienteering group, or a running group. And if you have retired to a new community and don't know anyone, join an exercise group. If you aren't spending enough time with your best friend, you can call her or him up and play a set of tennis. Make sure you talk about your lives while you play. Or if you aren't spending enough time with your kids, take a bike ride with them or take their bikes to the track and let them ride while you walk or jog. Also, fitness programs exist for parents and children.

Finally, consider how exercise relates to your spiritual need, desires such as searching for truth, meaning, and purpose; demonstrating respect and compassion for the good of others; sensing hope and optimism for self and others; and connecting to a larger reality.

Spirituality has important long-term health ramifications. Some Harvard researchers found that just watching films of people doing good deeds strengthens the viewers' immune system. A study of 2,700 people in Michigan found that the people who volunteered lived longer than those who didn't. Spirituality plays an important role in Dr. Dean Ornish's ongoing Lifestyle Heart Trial, which has been shown to reverse coronary artery disease in its participants. Along with quitting smoking, exercising regularly, and relying on a low-fat diet, participants are encouraged to develop faith, hope, and commitment in relation to a larger worldview.

Meanwhile, several psychologists have suggested that being strong spiritually may determine whether we pursue healthful behaviors. Carol Ryff of the University of Wisconsin at Madison and Burton Singer of Princeton University write, "It is individuals with positive purpose who are likely to sustain practices of taking care of themselves. Simply put, taking good care of oneself in terms of daily health practices presupposes a life that is worth taking care of."

So you can look at the physical-spiritual link in two ways. First, by developing a sense of purpose, a life's mission, you will be more likely to want to exercise, eat right, and so forth. Many books and resources can help you become more spiritual through techniques such as meditation and prayer, finding the beliefs that are best for you, and creating mission statements.

On the flip side, to help you become an Intrinsic Exerciser, use movement to help build and develop your spirituality. In his metaphor of the Runner, Sheehan alludes to the Inergy of exercise and enhancing one's spirit: "Running [becomes] a search for meaning, the run's fascinating meanderings in the interstices of the mind. The sights and sounds and touches of an entire life, the subconscious ready to harvest, make every run a treasure and a delight."

Once you are in tune with the exercise-spirituality connection, you'll begin to explore it more attentively. You can use movement to explore your own spirituality; running in a marathon or simply taking a walk, for example, can help you meditate on the natural world and forces beyond yourself.

One way to connect exercise with your spirituality is to consider the bigger picture of life. With running, for example, many beginners join the Leukemia and Lymphoma Society's Team in Training to prepare for a marathon. Gina Simile, of Modesto, California, joined a Team in Training group for her first marathon, raised pledges, and ran in the race. "You know, sometimes you think you can't take another step," she says, "and then you think about what these people went through." Other ways to enhance spirituality are to exercise outside occasionally to reestablish your connection with nature; to work out with all your senses to open you up to all the wonders of moving your body; and to help someone who is just starting to exercise. By giving something back, such as giving yourself up to that person for 20 or 30 minutes, you will get a spiritual boost. And gyms are popping up across the country that emphasize the exercise-spirituality connection.

Despite my breaking Inergy into four components, please remember that this is an artificial separation. The most powerful inner exercise experience is when you inergize exercise with your mental, social, and spiritual needs simultaneously.

Inergy Exercisers

My personal observations and experiences, conversations with regular exercisers, and readings of interviews conducted by my colleague Sue Jackson have led me to conclude that one of the things that people who maintain exercise do is practice Inergy consistently. One of the best examples comes from Kelly.

In January 1993, Kelly was a shy, self-affirmed couch potato and cigarette smoker. She was bored with her job and had little confidence. She had never been an athlete or participated in any sports at all, even though members of her family were athletes. In November, a friend suggested that she enter a local 5K road race. She had a simple goal: finish without walking. Kelly accomplished that goal and became hooked on racing immediately. The camaraderie of the other runners and the friendships she developed going to races were new to her. She started going to races every weekend so she could enjoy her new friendships and meet other people. She quit smoking about a year later, when she became more serious about her running. Kelly's confidence started to rise as a result of being able to run regularly. Being in good shape and meeting new friends helped her overcome her shyness.

Now Kelly feels like a different person. "I feel more confident and more in control of my life," she says. "I had suppressed the competitive side of me for so long. Now I run for all kinds of reasons, but the social and mental parts of it are really big for me. The confidence I've gained from running has carried over to every other part of my life." She has also told me that "I feel that there are a lot of people out there like me — people who were nonathletic and afraid to try. I like to tell my story because I think that if people hear it they will think, 'If she can do it, so can I.' I hope that people who know my story will realize that you don't have to be a high school or college superstar or have an athletic background to move your body. I did not start exercising until I was 32 years old. It's never too late, and now running is an integral part of my daily routine."

In February 2000, Kelly finished seventeenth in the U.S. Olympic Women's Marathon Trials held in Columbia, South Carolina, and she is now an elite marathon runner.

Chances are you will not become an elite exerciser, but you can apply the same strategies Kelly did to become a regular one. An Intrinsic Exerciser knows how to integrate his or her physical activity with other areas and needs in life. Consider a woman I'll call Cheryl, a 48-year-old swimmer. She is an example of an exercise maintainer who has used her swimming in an inergistic way. At the age of 34, Cheryl developed a serious back injury; she had no previous experience with swimming and was deathly afraid of the water. Her doctors said that swimming was the best activity for her, so, despite her fear, she paddled around the shallowest part of a nearby pool. Then she moved up to kickboards, learning the freestyle and backstroke, doing laps by herself, and becoming a competitive masters swimmer.

Focusing on how her exercise connects with her mental need, Cheryl says:

> Swimming has provided me with a sense of motivation to explore new things. . . . It's as though I've become a seeker of knowledge, and the more knowledge I have, I get the feeling that it makes it easier for me to cope with all the things that happen within my life. It's the sense of peacefulness that I have now, whereas I used to tear myself apart and worry over things. That's not to say I still don't fear things, but I do deal with them in a different way. . . . I believe my success in my professional life has come from my skill and mental attitude that I've developed in the pool.

Here's another example, from a 31-year-old swimmer — call him Brian — who also inergizes exercise with his mental need. He says:

> Swimming has helped me find the discipline to deal with all the emotional aspects of my life. It all blends together in some way or form . . . it has given me a lot more self-confidence, the sense that if I set my goals on something, not even swimming related, I know I can get it. That's one of the things that swimming has done for me.

Other Intrinsic Exercisers have discussed combining their physical activity with their mental and social needs. An 81-year-old cyclist who travels to various senior competitions explains: "My cycling has given me a broader outlook on life because I meet people who have different lifestyles. It's an education to see how other people are living." And Bill Gaston, president of the Van Cortlandt Track Club in the Bronx, says that when he runs with what he thinks is a good group, he experiences a "group glide" in which he feels in sync with the other runners.

Here's a story about exercise connecting to a spiritual element. Frank Roberts, of Fairfax, Virginia, wrote to me a couple of years ago after he read one of my articles. He congratulated me and attached an article he had written, "The Grieving Runner." In the article he described taking a run around a nearby lake while his wife was slowly dying of cancer. During the run Frank cried. He let go. He cried some more. He became depressed. But as he ran, he started to recognize the roots of his "dark, dank morbidity." He had been feeling guilty about his "selfish pleasure" while loved ones were suffering. But on that run he started to question these feelings: "What possible good to wife, self, or humanity could come of my suffering?" he writes. "The chronic stress of unalleviated depression (not the relief of grief fully expressed) could only threaten my own health, both mental and physical. Perhaps I would even begin to resent her for 'making me depressed,' which would subtly sabotage my ability to care for her."

Frank's run gave him time to think and realize this different perspective. He writes, "I realized that if I had not carved out this hunk of time for this 'selfish' pursuit — if I had locked myself into my schedule of 'shoulds' on my long list — I would not have made these discoveries, nor fully enjoyed this precious present moment. I ran on."

Frank ends his article with these thoughts: "So I leave my speculations and return to where they are inevitably leading me — to this path around this lake at this particular moment, which will never come again. And I realize with gratefulness that running's gift to me is more than health, it is sanity. On a run my thoughts and feelings have their presence and their passing. At 65, I do not run for records, even personal records. I run for the sake of my soul/body — and that fills me with such abundance that it overflows — and those lucky ones and friends can soak up the excess. So come join me in the feast of life. But first, a little run, O.K.?"

As you can see from these stories, anyone can learn to inergize exercise. Here is a three-step Inergy Plan that will help you connect your exercise with your mental, social, and spiritual needs:

1. Identify the most pressing mental, social, and spiritual needs in your life right now.

2. Determine ways in which moving your body can help you meet your need in each of the three areas.

3. Set one goal for each of three weeks that describes how you will connect your exercise with each of your needs. If three goals are too many for you, start with your most significant need and work on that for a while. Later, work on the two remaining ones.

8

....

Applying the Intrinsic Exerciser Mindset in Everyday Life

> That those things you call hardships and accursed, are, in the first place, for the good of the persons themselves to whom they come.
>
> — Lucius Annaeus Seneca, *Moral Essays*

Even though you now know — and practice — the four steps to intrinsic exercise, and have begun to pursue regular physical activity from the inside out, you will certainly face some situations that could bump you off the inner path. After all, Doug Newburg has found that most great performers face countless obstacles to living their lives as they want to. But he also found that world-class performers are very good at replacing their initial negative thoughts about a barrier with positive ones. This process helps them reenergize, remind them of why they are doing the activity. This boost of energy helps them to reattack the barrier, solve the problem, and creatively overcome or avoid any and all obstacles in their way.

Newburg calls this approach "your response to the response." All of us have an initial response to doing something new or challenging. For many beginning exercisers, their first response to the thought of exercising is a negative feeling or thought; if they hang on to it, it will only sabotage their desire to move. If this describes you, you must replace this initial, negative response with one that is positive and facilitating. The idea is:

Thought ➡	Response ➡	Response to the Response
Maybe I should exercise	People will laugh	I love the beauty and ritual of [my chosen exercise activity]. What do I care if people laugh? I laugh in the face of embarrassment — ha, ha, ha!

As an Intrinsic Exerciser, you can view vision, mastery, flow, and inergy as steps in building mental and emotional energy (positive responses to your response), enabling you to overcome the barriers that deter other people from exercising.

For example, you will probably find out that weather affects how often you exercise. During the winter in many places, people reduce their frequency of exercise because it's more challenging to move your body outdoors. Here is how one Intrinsic Exerciser has used a form of exerimaging to break through that barrier. Liz Harvey is a cyclist who lives in central California, which gets quite hot in the summer. She says, "I hate (hate!) to cycle in the heat but . . . I started to see myself as a cyclist who loves the heat. I visualized from the inside of my muscles loving to move in this intense heat and then moving as if lubricated by melted butter! . . . . With lots of water and Gatorade I actually enjoyed the ride on this past Sunday, even with the hill climbing in full sun."

Face it: most of the time you will not exercise under ideal weather conditions. Of course, you shouldn't exercise outside if it won't be safe. But you can use bad weather to enjoy your exercise even more than usual. Orlick has a simple technique he calls "channel changing" — clicking from a negative thought (ugh! it's raining) to a positive one (I love to splash in the puddles). Walking into strong winds? *Click*. "It will make me tough." Colder than normal? *Click*. "So this is what it's like to be a polar bear."

Another technique is to have an alternate plan for working out inside when the weather is really bad. Preparation is the key. I use my wife's stationary bike on days when it is safer to exercise indoors, for instance.

Injuries also affect your ability and motivation to exercise. The most emotional conversations I've had with people as I go around the country involve how injuries have wreaked havoc on their exercise routine. One day you are cruising along, healthy and able to move easily. The next day you are in a car accident and end up finding that parts of you hurt all the time.

But don't wallow in self-pity and what might have been. Instead, ask a medical professional how you can have as active a lifestyle as possible now. Consider the case of Anita Anderson.

Anita was a very active exerciser. While she was sitting at a stoplight, an oversize truck going 45 miles an hour rear-ended her car. After teaching an average of six aerobics classes a week, doing strength training, and competing in triathlons, Anita could no longer do any impact exercises — none. After six months of therapy three times a week, she decided to try her previous routine. After many unsuccessful attempts, she felt defeated and betrayed by her own body. She did not feel like the same person. Few of her friends understood. They would say, "You look fine. What's the big deal?" She wasn't fine. She missed the fatigue, the soreness, the rush after a great race or an intense aerobics class. It took a while, but Anita came to grips with the notion that she was not going to be able to exercise the way she used to. Now she bikes, walks, swims, and tries to maintain some level of fitness, knowing that as long as she's doing something physical, she is much happier.

As I've found with other people who have been hurt or slowed by injuries, Anita Anderson went through a period of trial and error — both physically and mentally — trying to come up with an approach that fit her physical challenge and her style. She continues to identify with exercise but in a different way. This may be the biggest hurdle of all for anyone who was a regular exerciser and now must exercise differently because of an injury. They think, "Why bother with exercise if I can't do what I'm used to doing? If I can't perform as well as I used to, then I'm just not going to exercise." One of the reasons many people stay in this "why bother" mental and emotional stage is that they can't let go of the exerciser they used to be. They had many goals and dreams, and now because of an injury they won't ever be achieved. This is where the Intrinsic Exerciser mindset shift becomes very important. People in this stage are seeing their past exercise from an Outside-In perspective, what it was giving them in the way of outcomes. They must get past that. The Intrinsic Exerciser attitude helps you find the joy in any movement you are doing right now.

Even if you don't suffer from an injury, you are going to face barriers if you want to exercise. You may love to spend your free time watching television, using a computer, reading, or just resting in between life events (which the time management guru David Allen calls "weird time"). In these cases, you can try to cut down one period of time — such as a half hour — spent on any of these activities. Be heartened: research shows that many people are most bored when watching TV but experience the most fun when playing sports and other physical games.

And if you have a child, think of your role as a model. New studies reveal that kids spend about 35 hours a week watching TV or using the computer — some 5 hours a day. You have an obligation to yourself and your child to use technology responsibly. You must ingrain in your child that doing something physical, such as shooting baskets together, is actually great fun. (It really is more enjoyable than watching a basketball game on television or playing basketball on a computer, although you may offer such virtual games as a catalyst to get your kid interested in doing the real thing).

Fortunately, as you become an Intrinsic Exerciser, you find that working on barriers to moving your body takes just a little energy and creativity. Usually, you face a point every day when you have to decide whether you want to exercise that day. Recognize that you will have to make this decision constantly — and that you must control it. At the beginning of each week, you should consider two possible barriers that interfere with your exercise routine that week. Next, develop and write down strategies to overcome those barriers.

Now is the time you may also want to investigate joining a health and fitness center. To find one that will actually help you exercise using the Intrinsic Exerciser philosophy, start with a tour of the possible facility at the time you think you will be there. Observe the people who are exercising and note how crowded it is. Look at whether people who look like you are exercising.

Also, see how many of the staff are available at any time. The most important ingredient in your success will be the staff-member ratio. And get a feel for the staff. You will do better if you develop a connection with a knowledgeable, caring professional. Make sure that the staff does not seem more concerned with their own fitness than their clients'.

Also, talk with the fitness director about your personal interests. (Make sure that the facility has such a person.) And be careful that the center does not focus only on programs from an Outside-In approach, such as losing weight.

Ask whether, if you join, you will be assigned a personal coach — or whether you must pay extra for personal attention. Such personal trainers are fine, but that should not be the only way to get help and attention in a facility. Aid should be part of your membership. Also ask about special programs for beginners. You want a facility that offers programs to fit your needs. You are not just another sheep being herded into the barn.

If you haven't exercised much, you probably never quite know what to do with your mind before, during, and afterward — whether to distract your mind from your body or tune in to your body. To maximize your enjoyment in the long term, learn to do both.

Much of the health and fitness profession assumes that distraction is central to keeping people exercising. This strategy is often useful to get you started. Then, as your body gets used to moving, tune in periodically. And as you get more experienced, develop more advanced strategies to keep tuning in.

Distractions that I consider okay include television, reading, or even surfing the Internet. The more you enjoy the distraction, the better. The number-one complaint by health and fitness center members concerns a lack of variety in the music, TV, magazines, and the like. Therefore, many centers surround you with distraction, such as offering headphones for watching health and wellness educational programs or listening to your favorite music. And virtual reality exercise equipment allows you to experience many worlds as you pedal or climb. A color monitor displays the visual effects along with the music.

Music is the old standby, of course, for it seems to have a

more powerful effect on the mind and body than other distractions. Research indicates that music helps the exerciser pay less attention to bodily sensations and elevates mood, especially during moderate- to high-intensity exercise. Music also enhances the rhythm of an exerciser's movement. Consider aerobics classes without music. But recognize that exercise physiologists have found that exposure to noise above 108 decibels — the noise level of a blow dryer — during exercise results in temporary hearing loss, and repeated exposures at that level can lead to permanent hearing loss. Most music during exercise is above that level. If you use music as a major form of distraction, turn it down for your own good. Also, the music may push you to work out too vigorously and cause an injury.

A final word of caution: use distraction techniques only at low to moderate intensities of exercise. Some sport and exercise psychology research shows that distraction at high levels of intensity can also put you at risk for injury.

Ralph LaForge, a leading mind-body exercise expert at Duke University, recommends that as you learn to tune in to your body, practice some basic tuning-in strategies before and after your exercise. For example, during your warm-up you can perform a nonjudgmental mental check of your body. Focus on various parts of your body. Think about how your face feels. Feel whether your stomach or legs are tight. You will also find that simply being aware of your breathing pattern before and after exercise will connect your mind with your body.

Similar to their use before and after exercise, tuning-in strategies used during exercise should be brief, at least initially. A good rule of thumb is to start with two or three body scans for every 30 minutes of exercise and build up to five. Just for fun, switch from tuning out to tuning in at varying points, even if only for a minute or two.

As you advance, I recommend that you keep a journal to record your mental and physical reactions during training and racing sessions. Visualize your ideal performance state and use feedback forms. You can develop mini-feedback forms completed immediately after a performance. These forms can address a variety of mind-body connections, such as anxiety levels, concentration, and physiological functioning.

The End of the Beginning

As you have read this book — and tried some of the activities — you should be starting to think and feel a little differently about your exercise experiences. That's good. You have begun the mindset transformation — from Outside-In to Inside-Out — that is so crucial to enjoying exercise.

To stay on the inner path of the Intrinsic Exerciser, you should ask yourself these questions periodically:

- Do I see myself as an exerciser, and how do I want my movement to feel? (Vision)

- Do I base my feelings of exercise success on my own criteria? (Mastery)

- Do I get into it when I move my body? (Flow)

- Do I connect exercise with my other life needs? (Inergy)

129

No one can turn you into an Intrinsic Exerciser. I can only guide you to the inner path. You are the one who must travel that road. The questions will serve as your intrinsic light to the joyful path that movement can bring. Ask them of yourself when you feel you are swerving off the path or can't find your way. They will keep you an Inside-Out exerciser.

Epilogue

It was a dreary Saturday in March — drizzly, damp, and cold. One of those days you often experience in the Midwest in the lull just before spring. My family was settled in for the afternoon. I was dragging, a little fatigued from the week's activities. I knew it was time to go for a run. I wasn't overly enthusiastic about going out, but I did. My goal was to let my body take me where it wanted to go. No pressure, no time goals. This was an experience run. I started down the hill on my normal course but soon veered off and headed toward our old neighborhood. I passed a man running alongside his daughter, who was riding her bike. We waved as we passed. The daughter had the biggest smile I'd ever seen. I copied her smile for a couple of minutes. It felt good. I descended a hill that passed over a creek. The rain had caused the creek to swell. The sound of the fast-running water spurred me to move faster up the approaching hill. For some reason, I was focused on the sound the wind was making as it hit my face. I had never heard that sound before. It was kind of like a *whoosh, whoosh*. It was a lovely sound.

Then I was at our old house. It seemed in disrepair. This saddened me, so I moved quickly past it, nearing the turn-around point. I looked up, and these giant spruce trees were whipping in the wind. They seemed so ominous. On the way back, a funny little dog decided to join me for a while. I spurted and then slowed down. I did this a few times, playing with the dog until it became bored and dropped back. After that, my mindset changed. I picked up the pace. I felt loose. I turned the corner to head up the hill that would bring me back home. My goal now was to run hard, run strong. Concentrate. Focus. I imagined I was Walter "Sweetness" Payton, the great Chicago Bear running back who passed away a few years ago. I heard stories that he used to run up hills as part of his training. I avoided tacklers. I ran like Sweetness. I crested the hill and turned onto my flat road. I jogged the eighth of a mile to my house. I stopped my watch — 41:00. The time struck me, as it matched my age at the time. I cooled down by walking back and forth on our sidewalk. My daughter and I once came up with an idea for a children's story about a sidewalk. "I've got to write that story," I thought. I savored each breath that returned me to my relaxed state. I walked into the house. Life was pretty much the same as when I had gone out for the run. But I felt different. I had this inner glow that could only have come from being an Intrinsic Exerciser. It stayed with me for the rest of the day.

Every exercise session you participate in gives you an opportunity to get closer to the ultimate Intrinsic Exerciser, to release and experience the spontaneous joy in moving your body. Embracing the mindset of an Intrinsic Exerciser leads to an ongoing process of self-discovery and self-expression. Joy can always be found in the exercise experience when you find meaning in it, when you base your success on your own criteria, when you find a way to stay in the moment, and when you connect your need to move with your other needs in life.

Of course, barriers and obstacles will arise. Embrace them with your mind, body, and spirit. Be creative with your solutions. The answer is found within. Don't be afraid to tune in to your body. It wants to move. Listen to the inner voice that will make any movement experience an intrinsic one. As you begin to remove the extrinsic layers of Outside-In — reduction in risk of disease, information overload, and looking to the future — you will begin to uncover the mover that has always been there, waiting to be unleashed.

Be ready for your Intrinsic Exerciser and then let it out. You will experience your body and the world in ways that are natural, wonderful, and joyful.

Welcome home.

Notes
Bibliography

Notes

Introduction

3 "You may be a little": Kuczmarski et al. (1994).

1. Outside-In: The Extrinsic Approach to Exercise

9 "Those who cannot change their minds": From an article by Peter Townsley in *AWHP's Worksite Health* (1996, p. 47). I have been unable to locate the original source.

10 If the Outside-In approach worked: Mokdad et al. (1999), (2001).

10 Billions of dollars on weight-loss products: Begley (1991).

10 "This dramatic new evidence": McClam (2001).

10 Approximately 300,000 Americans: McGinnis and Foege (1993).

11 "The message is out there": McClam (2001).

12 Behavior change approaches: See Mitchell (1988) and Dreyfus and Dreyfus (1986) for fuller explanations about why our present society is dominated by rationalization.

12 "Successfully changing our sedentary society": Pate et al. (1995, p. 405).

12 "We know that if everybody": Gorman (2001, p. 57).

13 only about one of five people exercise regularly: U.S. Department of Health and Human Services (1996).

14 "The only thing you need to do": Miller (2000, p. 58).

15 50 to 75 percent . . . drop out: Dishman (1988).

17 Other changes in family life: U.S. House of Representatives, Committee on Ways and Means (1998).

17 "Within households": Haskell (1996, p. S-39).

18 "The expectation has been": Haskell (1996, p. S-39).

18 Simply put, work: Bridges (1994). The U.S. Commerce Department's Census Bureau reports that women owned 5.4 million companies — most of them considered small businesses — in 1997, a 16 percent rise from 5 years earlier. Reported in the *Baltimore Sun* by Andrea Walker (2001). The Oxford Health Plans survey comes from *Business Wire* (2001). Alderman (1995).

18 The employees still in corporations: According to Robinson et al. (2000), "The U.S. has now passed Japan as the industrialized world's most overworked land — Americans average a paltry nine days off after the first year on the job."

19 Paradoxically, the research: See Pelletier (1991) and Shephard (1999) for thorough reviews of this literature. Hong (2000). Langer (1989).

19 Based on what is going on: Rippe (1989). Dishman et al. (1985).

21 "The secret to getting people": Maddux (1997, p. 342).

2. Inside-Out: The Intrinsic Approach to Exercise

23 "Change — real change": Covey (1989, p. 317).

24 "I couldn't care less": Fraser (MODE, 1999, p. 128).

24 "I believe in living an active life": Beech (1998, p. 13).

25 "you can take the person out of the Stone Age": Nicholson (1998, p. 135).

25 "These changes constitute": Bortz (1985, p. 150).

25 Our brains have evolved: Gage's thoughts come from an article on the Internet by the *Times*'s science writer Robert Lee Hotz (1999). Gage was featured in *Time* by Park (2000) as an innovator in neurobiology. For the mouse study, see Van Praag et al. (1999), and for the adult brain study, see Kempermann and Gage (1999).

26 "Our abilities to run": Heinrich (2000, p. 76).

27 "We are biologically equipped": From an unpublished book chapter by Pat Eisenman (1996), an exercise physiologist at the University of Utah.

28 *I used to live:* The basis for the story comes from the research on intrinsic motivation by Mark Lepper and David Greene and is summarized in *The Hidden Costs of Reward* (1978). The point of the story is relevant to the discussion about Outside-In and Inside-Out.

30 Consider this chart: This figure is adapted from one used by my colleague Robin Vealey in a course on motivation. A more scientific version appears in Deci and Ryan (2000, p. 237).

31 Motivational scientists also suggest: A thorough description of the three kinds of intrinsic motivation appears in Vallerand (1997).

32 To know, to accomplish: According to Deci and Ryan (1987), self-determination is characterized by autonomous initiation and regulation and reflects a true expression of oneself. They assume that the more one's behavior is intrinsically motivated, the greater will be his or her self-determination.

33 Here is a quiz: The quiz includes one item from the Exercise Motivation Scale, which measures each of the eight kinds of exercise motivation. Fuzhong Li, an exercise scientist at the Oregon Research Institute, developed the Exercise Motivation Scale. A more complete description can be found in Li (1999).

34 A study at the University of Texas: Intrinsic motivation also extends beyond exercise. A study by Susan Curry of the University of Washington and her colleagues evaluated intrinsic and extrinsic motivation interventions with smoking cessation. As you can figure out by now, financial incentive had no effect on long-term cessation rates. Intrinsically oriented, personal feedback increased the use of materials and was associated with higher rates of smoking cessation 3 months after the materials were distributed to both users and nonusers of the program.

34 Overall, Inside-Out: These sources appeared in the YMCA of Canada's weekly Marketing E-Lab report (1996).

35 "The fact is that few people": Sheehan (1983, p. 160).

Notes

36 "Play returns us": Sheehan (1983, p. 161).
36 "sport makes us fully functioning": Sheehan (1983, p. 161).
37 Surveys show: Kraus (1994).
38 When I look back: The names of most of these games are self-explanatory. But sock 'em soccer was kicking the ball at your opponent rather than shooting at a goal; pickle ball is a baseball adaptation of monkey in the middle; and infield used half of the baseball diamond and was played when we didn't have enough kids for a full-blown baseball game.
39 Strauss's interview: Strauss and Miller (2001).
40 I realize that the notion: Several studies reviewed by Csikszentmihalyi (1997) show that when people are at work, they say they wish they were doing something else more than at any other time of the day. Also, a *USA Today* article by Stephanie Armour (1999) cited numerous experts about the problem of boredom in the workplace.

3. The Intrinsic Exerciser: An Overview

41 "One is alive": Allen and Fahey (1977, p. 112).
42 "We have the unique ability": Heinrich (2000, p. 74).
43 "Clearly, enjoyment": Massimini et al. (1988, p. 60).
45 The last step is: A number of wellness models typically outline a variety of needs — physical, social, mental, emotional, intellectual, and environmental — but I like Stephen Covey's simplified approach in *First Things First*. Like wellness advocates, Covey suggests that each of us has four basic needs — physical, mental, social, and spiritual — and that not meeting any one of these needs reduces the quality of life. Many of us recognize these needs but tend to see them as separate compartments of life. Covey emphasizes the connection among them. My approach is to take the physical component and show you how to connect it to the other needs.
46 "There can no longer be any doubt": Adler (1938, p. 68).

4. Step 1: Activate the Intrinsic Exerciser with Vision

53 "What we can do": Glasser (1990, p. 87).
56 "We tend to act": Sonstroem (1997, p. 19).
56 "Possible selves": Markus and Nurius (1986, p. 954).

Notes

57 "If the self includes": Csikszentmihalyi (1993, p. 217).

59 "Of all the ways": Bingham (1999, p. 177). Bingham transformed his life by becoming a regular exerciser. I highly recommend his *Courage to Start* as another source of inspiration for the Intrinsic Exerciser.

65 Resonance developed out of interviews: Doug Newburg has interviewed world-class performers, such as the three-time Olympic Gold medalist swimmer Jeff Rouse and the Grammy Award–winner Bruce Hornsby, to uncover the secrets of living a meaningful life and being a top performer. I am quite fortunate to have been introduced to the whole idea of resonance.

66 "Although it may be difficult": Ravizza (1977, p. 102).

68 Start by making simple observations: For example, see Gallwey's *Inner Game of Tennis* (1997, rev. ed.).

69 As you become more aware: The latest trend is for exercise scientists to advocate the lifestyle approach on the assumption that it is easier for most people to incorporate physical activity into their daily routine than it is to perform the traditional, structured recommendations. I'm not totally convinced; you still need to have the desire to move to become more physically active. I sometimes think the structured approach gives people what they want and is no more difficult in the long run than the lifestyle approach.

71 "During my high school days": Kristi's story originally appeared as part of an exam question I asked graduate students.

73 "Now there's one way to change": Walsch (1996, p. 167).

74 "It's important now": Walsch (1996, p. 168).

77 "The most powerful imagery": Orlick (1998, p. 73).

77 "It is through looking back": Wong (1995, p. 34).

5. Step 2: Stay on Track with Mastery

80 "Our current society": Leonard (1991, p. 4).

81 According to motivational theorists: Many good sources in sport and exercise psychology research explain these two views of achievement and success. See Roberts (1992) as an example.

82 People with low ability: For example, see Jackson and Roberts (1992).

83 The mastery folks responded to exercise: Duda et al. (1990).

141

84 Don't underestimate the power: See Hart et al. (1989) for a fuller scientific explanation of physique anxiety.

85 Rita Callahan: I interviewed Rita in July 1997 at the Mission Valley YMCA in San Diego.

86 One of the best ways: I originally interviewed Stacy Wegley and Tony Poggiali for an article that appeared in *IDEA Health and Fitness Source* (2000).

88 "I have never encountered": Orlick (1986, p. 10).

88 Mastery guides you: Kimiecik et al. (1990).

89 Here's what one: These quotes from masters athletes come from transcripts of interviews conducted by Susan Jackson at the 1994 World Masters Games in Brisbane, Australia. I greatly appreciate Jackson's permission to use them here.

90 The effects of mastery on experience: See Dempsey, Kimiecik, and Horn (1993), Kimiecik, Horn, and Shurin (1996), and Kimiecik and Horn (1998).

91 You need to tread lightly: Ryan and Deci (2000), Dishman (1987).

92 "noted that when she gave herself": Bain et al. (1989, p. 142).

6. Step 3: Stay in the Moment with Flow

96 "Flow is a source": Csikszentmihalyi (1997, p. 140).

97 "It's like real high": Both quotes come from participants in research studies, so I'm keeping them anonymous. The first, from a runner, is from an interview conducted by Chris Szabo, a former graduate student at Miami University. See Szabo and Kimiecik (1997); the second, from a triathlete, is from an interview conducted by Susan Jackson.

98 Flow, which is a hot topic: These flow characteristics have become universal and can be found in almost any article or book on flow. See Kimiecik and Stein (1992) or Jackson and Csikszentmihalyi (1999).

99 Second, the merging of action and awareness: See Jackson (1992) for plenty of examples from elite athletes.

100 "exercising control in difficult situations": Csikszentmihalyi (1997, p. 129).

102 In other words, mastery: Csikszentmihalyi and Schneider (2000).

104 Many people who focus on losing weight: The National

Weight Control Registry (800-606-NWCR) was founded in 1993 by Dr. James Hill and Dr. Rena Wing. It is not a treatment program but rather a national database that identifies a large group of people who have been successful at maintaining substantial weight loss over a long time.

105 Joann Donnelly: I originally interviewed Joann for an article that was published in *IDEA Health and Fitness Source* (2000).

105 If all else fails: George Blackburn, one of the nation's top obesity doctors, suggested 10,000 steps in a *USA Today* article by Nanci Hellmich (2000).

106 Self-Guided Flow Form: This form is adapted from the Experiential Sampling Method (ESM) that Csikszentmihalyi has used in most of his research on flow.

7. Step 4: Fuel the Physical Fire with Inergy

108 "The ultimate reality": Smuts (1961, p. 117).

110 "Positive psychological benefits": Plante (1999, p. 292).

110 A study by Robert Motl: Csikszentmihalyi (1997, pp. 136–37) talks about reflecting on life when in a positive mood from a flow perspective. I suggest that after exercise — if you are into it — would be as good a time as any. Some people do this during exercise.

111 Next, consider our social needs: A number of studies have consistently supported the relationship between social support and exercise as indicated in *Physical Activity and Health: A Report of the Surgeon General*, Department of Health and Human Services (1996).

111 "I know now that there are": Bingham (1999, p. 166).

112 Research repeatedly shows: Uchino et al. (1996).

113 Spirituality has important: Growald and Lusks (1988) and Ornish (1990).

114 "It is individuals with positive purpose": Ryff and Singer (1998, p. 22).

114 "Running [becomes] a search": Sheehan (1983, p. 160).

115 "You know, sometimes you think": Moore (1999, p. C3).

116 In January 1993: I found out about Kelly in a letter she wrote in *Runner's Spotlite* (February 1998). I interviewed her by phone that summer.

118 "Swimming has provided me with": Cheryl and Brian are pseudonyms for two masters athletes interviewed by Susan Jackson at the 1994 World Masters Games.
118 "My cycling has given me": From an interview by Susan Jackson.
119 "group glide": From a *New York Times* article by Nancy Stedman (1999, p. D7).
119 Here's a story about: Roberts's article "The Grieving Runner" was first published in the *American Medical Athletic Association Journal*.

8. Applying the Intrinsic Exerciser Mindset in Everyday Life

121 "That those things you call hardships": Seneca, in *Moral Essays*, in *The Problem of Evil*, Mark Larrimore, ed. (2001, p. 20).
122 "your response to the response": Newburg's understanding of performance has helped me immeasurably to help others with the "response to the response" approach to overcoming obstacles to exercise and, more important, to living a purposeful life. I accept full blame for any errors in translating his views.
122 "I hate (hate!) to cycle": I received this story from Liz, who is part of the Intrinsic Exerciser e-mail group.
123 Face it: most of the time: I originally read about the *Click* approach in Orlick (1996).
124 Anita was a very active: Anita sent me her story via e-mail.
125 "weird time": Hammonds (2000).
125 Be heartened: Csikszentmihalyi (1997).
125 And if you have a child: This estimate comes from a Kaiser Family Foundation survey reported by Peter Johnson in *USA Today* (1999).
127 Music is the old: Karageorghis and Terry (1997). The decibel level guidelines are based on an interview with Helaine Alessio, an exercise physiologist at Miami University who studies the relationships among exercise, fitness, and hearing.
128 Ralph LaForge: I interviewed Ralph for an article that appeared in *IDEA Health and Fitness Source* (1999).

Bibliography

Adler, A. 1938. *Social interest: A challenge to mankind*. London: Faber and Faber.

Alderman, L. February 1995. Here comes the four-income family. *Money*, 149–55.

American Sports Data, Inc. 1996. *A comprehensive study of lifestyle, physical fitness and the health club experience in the U.S.*

Armour, S. May 21, 1999. Boredom drains workers, workforce. *USA Today*, 12B.

Bain, L., Wilson, T., and Chaikand, E. 1989. Participant perceptions of exercise programs for overweight women. *Research Quarterly for Exercise and Sport*, 60, 134–43.

Becker, M. H. 1993. A medical sociologist looks at health promotion. *Journal of Health and Social Behavior*, 34, 1–6.

Beech, M. Aug. 24, 1998. Bill Rodgers, marathoner. *Sports Illustrated*, 13.

Begley, C. 1991. Government should strengthen regulation in the weight loss industry. *Journal of the American Dietetic Association*, 91, 1255–57.

Bingham, J. 1999. *The courage to start*. New York: Fireside.

Bortz, W. 1985. Physical exercise as an evolutionary force. *Journal of Human Evolution*, 14, 145–55.

Bibliography

Business Wire. February 2001. Online via NewsEdge Corporation.

Bridges, W. 1994. *JobShift*. Reading, Mass.: Addison-Wesley.

Brown, D., Wang, Y., Ward, A., Ebbeling, C., Fortlage, L., Puleo, E., Benson, H., and Rippe, J. 1995. Chronic psychological effects of exercise and exercise plus cognitive strategies. *Medicine and Science in Sports and Exercise, 27,* 765–75.

Covey, S. 1989. *The 7 habits of highly effective people.* New York: Fireside.

Covey, S., Merrill, A., and Merrill, R. 1994. *First things first.* New York: Simon and Schuster.

Csikszentmihalyi, M. 1990. *Flow: The psychology of optimal experience.* New York: Harper and Row.

———. 1993. *The evolving self.* New York: Harper and Row.

———. 1997. *Finding flow.* New York: HarperCollins.

Csikszentmihalyi, M., and Schneider, B. 2000. *Becoming adult: How teenagers prepare for the world of work.* New York: Basic Books.

Curry, S., Wagner, E., and Grothaus, L. 1991. Evaluation of intrinsic and extrinsic motivation interventions with a self-help smoking cessation program. *Journal of Consulting and Clinical Psychology, 59,* 318–24.

Deci, E., and Ryan, R. 1987. The support of autonomy and the control of behavior. *Journal of Personality and Social Psychology, 53,* 1024–37.

———. 2000. The "what" and "why" of goal pursuits: Human needs and self-determination of behavior. *Psychological Inquiry, 11,* 227–68.

———. 1985. *Intrinsic motivation and self-determination in human behavior.* New York: Plenum Press.

Dempsey, J., Kimiecik, J., and Horn, T. 1993. Parental influence on children's moderate-to-vigorous physical activity: An expectancy-value approach. *Pediatric Exercise Science, 5,* 151–67.

Dishman, R. 1987. Exercise adherence and habitual physical activity. In W. Morgan and S. Goldston, eds., *Exercise and mental health* (57–83). Washington, D.C.: Hemisphere.

Dishman, R., ed. 1988. *Exercise adherence: Its impact on public health.* Champaign, Ill.: Human Kinetics.

Dishman, R., and Buckworth, J. 1996. Increasing physical activity: A quantitative synthesis. *Medicine and Science in Sports and Exercise, 28,* 706–19.

Dishman, R., Sallis, J., and Orenstein, D. 1985. The determinants of physical activity and exercise. *Public Health Reports, 100,* 158–71.

Dreyfus, H., and Dreyfus, S. 1986. *Mind over machine: The power of human intuition and expertise in the era of the computer.* New York: Free Press.

Duda, J., Sedlock, D., et al. March 1990. *The influence of goal perspective on perceived exertion and affect ratings during submaximal exercise.* Paper presented at the annual meeting of the American Alliance for Health, Physical Education, Recreation, and Dance, New Orleans.

Dunn, A., Marcus, B., Kampert, J., et al. 1999. Comparison of lifestyle and structured interventions to increase physical activity and cardiorespiratory fitness: A randomized trial. *Journal of the American Medical Association, 281,* 327–34.

Eisenman, P. 1996. *Designed for movement: An evolutionary perspective.* Unpublished manuscript.

Ekkekakis, P., Hall, E., VanLanduyt, L., and Petruzello, S. 2000. *Journal of Behavioral Medicine, 23,* 245–75.

Erwin, K. 1996. *Group techniques for aging adults: Putting geriatric skills enhancement into practice.* Washington, D.C.: Taylor and Francis.

Fahey, B. 1977. The passionate body. In D. Allen and B. Fahey, eds., *Being human in sport* (pp. 111–19). Philadelphia: Lea and Febiger.

Field, L., and Steinhardt, M. 1992. The relationship of internally directed behavior to self-reinforcement, self-esteem, and expectancy values for exercise. *American Journal of Health Promotion, 7,* 21–27.

Fraser, L. April 1999. Exercise dilettante. *Mode, 128.*

Gallwey, T. 1997. *The inner game of tennis,* rev. ed. New York: Random House.

Gammage, K., Hall, C., and Rodgers, W. 2000. More about exercise imagery. *Sport Psychologist, 14,* 348–59.

Gauvin, L., Rejeski, W., and Reboussin, B. 2000. Contributions of acute bouts of vigorous physical activity to explaining diurnal variations in feeling states in active, middle-aged women. *Health Psychology, 19,* 365–75.

Bibliography

Glasser, W. 1990. *The quality school.* New York: HarperPerennial.

Gorman, C. Feb. 5, 2001. Repairing damage. *Time,* 52–58.

Growald, E., and Lusks, A. March 1988. Beyond self. *American Health,* 51–53.

Hammonds, K. May 2000. You can do anything — but not everything. *Fast Company* (online version), 2.

Hart, L., Leary, M., and Rejeski, W. 1989. The measurement of social physique anxiety. *Journal of Sport and Exercise Psychology, 11,* 94–104.

Haskell, W. 1996. Physical activity, sport, and health: Toward the next century. *Research Quarterly for Exercise and Sport, 67,* 37–47.

Hausenblas, H., Hall, C., Rodgers, W., and Munroe, K. 1999. Exercise imagery: Its nature and measurement. *Journal of Applied Sport Psychology, 11,* 171–80.

Heinrich, B. September 2000. Endurance predator. *OUTSIDE,* 70–76.

Hellmich, N. June 15, 2000. Doctors urged to get a grip on fat. *USA Today,* 10D.

Hong, S. 2000. Exercise and psychoneuroimmunology. *International Journal of Sport Psychology, 31,* 204–27.

Hooker, K., and Kaus, C. 1992. Possible selves and health behaviors in later life. *Journal of Aging and Health, 4,* 390–411.

Hotz, R. Feb. 23, 1999. Active mind, body linked to brain growth. Internet source.

Jackicic, J., Winters, C., Lang, W., and Wing, R. 1999. Effects of intermittent exercise and home exercise equipment on adherence, weight loss, and fitness in overweight women. *Journal of the American Medical Association, 282,* 1554–60.

Jackson, S. 1992. Athletes in flow: A qualitative investigation of flow states in elite figure skaters. *Journal of Applied Sport Psychology, 4,* 161–80.

Jackson, S., and Csikszentmihalyi, M. 1999. *Flow in sports: The keys to optimal experiences and performances.* Champaign, Ill.: Human Kinetics.

Jackson, S., and Roberts, G. 1992. Positive performance states of athletes: Toward a conceptual understanding of peak performance. *Sport Psychologist, 6,* 156–71.

Johnson, P. Feb. 18, 1999. TV grabs biggest share of kids' time. *USA Today,* D1.

Bibliography

Karageorghis, C., and Terry, P. 1997. The psychophysical effects of music in sport and exercise: A review. *Journal of Sport Behavior, 20,* 54–68.

Kempermann, G., and Gage, F. 1999. New nerve cells for the adult brain. *Scientific American, 280,* 48–53.

Kendzierski, D. 1990. Exercise self-schemata: Cognitive and behavioral correlates. *Health Psychology, 9,* 69–82.

Kendzierski, D., and DeCarlo, K. 1991. Physical activity enjoyment scale: Two validation studies. *Journal of Sport and Exercise Psychology, 13,* 50–64.

Kimiecik, J. March 1998. The path of the intrinsic exerciser. *IDEA Health and Fitness Source,* 34–42.

——. April 1999. Zooming in on attentional focus. *IDEA Health and Fitness Source,* 36–43.

——. March 2000. Bashing through barriers: How to help clients navigate their internal obstacle course to a lifetime of regular exercise. *IDEA Health and Fitness Source,* 39–46.

——. January/February 2000. Learn to love exercise. *Psychology Today, 20,* 22.

——. April 2000. The home run. *Runner's World,* 112.

Kimiecik, J., and Horn, T. 1998. Parental beliefs and children's moderate-to-vigorous physical activity. *Research Quarterly for Exercise and Sport, 69,* 163–75.

Kimiecik, J., Horn, T., and Shurin, C. 1996. Relationships among children's beliefs, perceptions of their parents' beliefs, and their moderate-to-vigorous physical activity. *Research Quarterly for Exercise and Sport, 67,* 324–36.

Kimiecik J., and Jackson, S. In press. Optimal experience in sport: A flow perspective. In T. Horn, ed., *Advances in Sport Psychology,* 2nd ed. Champaign, Ill.: Human Kinetics.

Kimiecik, J., Jackson, S., and Giannini, J. 1990. Striving for exercise goals: An examination of motivational orientations and exercise behavior in unsupervised joggers, swimmers, and cyclists. In L. Vander Velden and J. Humphrey, eds., *Psychology and Sociology of Sport: Current Selected Research,* Vol. II (17–32). New York: AMS Press.

Kimiecik, J., and Stein, G. 1992. Examining flow experiences in sport contexts: Conceptual issues and methodological concerns. *Journal of Applied Sport Psychology, 4,* 144–60.

King, A., Taylor, C. B., Haskell, W., and DeBusk, R. 1989. Influence of regular aerobic exercise on psychological health: A randomized, controlled trial of healthy middle-aged adults. *Health Psychology, 8,* 305–24.

Kraus, R. 1994. *Leisure in a changing America: Multicultural perspectives.* New York: Macmillan College Publishing.

Kuczmarski, R., Flegal, K., et al. 1994. Increasing prevalence of overweight among US adults. *Journal of the American Medical Association, 272,* 205–11.

Langer, E. 1989. *Mindfulness.* Reading, Mass.: Addison-Wesley.

Larrimore, M., ed. 2001. The problem of evil: A reader. Malden, Mass.: Blackwell.

Leonard, G. 1991. *Mastery: The keys to success and long-term fulfillment.* New York: Dutton.

Lepper, M., and Greene, D., eds. 1978. *The hidden costs of reward: New perspectives on the psychology of human motivation.* Hillsdale, N.J.: Lawrence Erlbaum.

Levine, J., Eberhardt, N., and Jensen, M. 1999. Role of nonexercise activity thermogenesis in resistance to fat gain in humans. *Science, 283,* 212–14.

Li, F. 1999. The exercise motivation scale: Its multifaceted structure and content validity, *Journal of Applied Sport Psychology, 11,* 97–115.

Maddux, J. 1997. Habit, health, and happiness. *Journal of Sport and Exercise Psychology, 19,* 331–46.

Mandigo, J., Thompson, L., and Couture, R. June 1998. *Equating flow theory with the quality of children's physical activity experiences.* Presented at the annual North American Psychology of Sport and Physical Activity Conference, St. Charles, Illinois.

Markus, H., and Nurius, P. 1986. *American Psychologist, 9,* 954–69.

Marinelli, R., and Plummer, O. 1999. Healthy aging: Beyond exercise. *Activities, adaptation, and aging, 23,* 1–11.

Martin, J., Dubbert, P., et al. 1984. Behavioral control of exercise in sedentary adults: Studies 1 through 6. *Journal of Consulting and Clinical Psychology, 52,* 795–811.

Massimini, F., Csikszentmihalyi, M., and Delle Fave, A. 1988. In Csikszentmihalyi, M., and Csikszentmihalyi, I., eds., *Optimal experience: Psychological studies of flow in consciousness* (364–83). New York: Cambridge University Press.

May, R. 1953. *Man's search for himself.* New York: W. W. Norton.

McAuley, E., Blissmer, B., et al. 2000. Social relations, physical

Bibliography

activity and well-being in older adults. *Preventive Medicine,* *31,* 608–17.

McAuley, E., Wraith, S., and Duncan, T. 1991. Self-efficacy, perceptions of success, and intrinsic motivation for exercise. *Journal of Applied Social Psychology, 21,* 139–55.

McClam, E. Jan. 26, 2001. CDC: Diabetes, obesity becoming epidemic. Associated Press (Internet source).

McGinnis, J., and Foege, W. 1993. Actual causes of death in the United States. *Journal of the American Medical Association, 270,* 2207–12.

Miller, G. January/February 2001. A brand-new start. *Cooking Light,* 58–64.

Mitchell, R. G. 1988. Sociological implications of the flow experience. In Csikszentmihalyi, M., and Csikszentmihalyi, I., eds., *Optimal experience: Psychological studies of flow in consciousness* (36–59). New York: Cambridge University Press.

Mokdad, A., Ford, E., et al. 2001. The continuing increase of diabetes in the U.S. *Diabetes Care, 24,* 412.

Mokdad, A., Serdula, M., et al. 1999. The spread of the obesity epidemic in the United States, 1991–1998. *Journal of the American Medical Association, 282,* 1519–22.

Moore, D. L. Oct. 22, 1999. Running's second wind. *USA Today,* 3C.

Motl, R., Berger, B., and Leuschen, P. 2000. The role of enjoyment in the exercise-mood relationship. *International Journal of Sport Psychology, 31,* 347–63.

Nicholson, N. July/August 1998. How hardwired is human behavior? *Harvard Business Review,* 135 47.

Orlick, T. 1986. *Psyching for sport.* Champaign, Ill.: Human Kinetics.

———. 1990. *In pursuit of excellence.* Champaign, Ill.: Human Kinetics.

———. 1998. *Embracing your potential.* Champaign, Ill.: Human Kinetics.

Ornish, D. 1990. *Dr. Dean Ornish's program for reversing heart disease.* New York: Ballantine.

Park, A. Aug. 7, 2000. Old brains, new tricks. *Time,* 70.

Pate, R., Blair, S., Haskell, W., et al. 1995. Physical activity and public health: A recommendation from the Centers for Disease Control and Prevention and the American College of

Bibliography

Sports Medicine. *Journal of the American Medical Association,* 273, 402–7.

Pelletier, K. 1991. A review and analysis of the health and cost-effective outcome studies of comprehensive health promotion and disease prevention programs. *American Journal of Health Promotion,* 5, 311–15.

Plante, T. 1999. Could the perception of fitness account for many of the mental and physical health benefits of exercise? *Advances in Mind-Body Medicine,* 15, 291–95.

Ravizza, K. 1977. The body unaware. In D. Allen and B. Fahey, eds., *Being human in sport* (99–109). Philadelphia: Lea and Febiger.

Reiss, S. January/February 2001. Secrets of happiness. *Psychology Today,* 50–56.

Rippe, J. 1996. *Fit over forty.* New York: Quill.

———. 1989. *Fit for success: Proven strategies for executive health.* New York: Prentice Hall.

Roberts, F. The grieving runner. *American Medical Athletic Association Journal.*

Roberts, G., ed. 1992. *Motivation in sport and exercise.* Champaign, Ill.: Human Kinetics.

Robinson, J., Walljasper, J., and Kumer, S. September/October 2000. *Utne Reader,* 48–54.

Ryan, R., and Deci, E. 2000. Self-determination theory and the facilitation of intrinsic motivation, social development, and well-being. *American Psychologist,* 55, 68–78.

Ryff, C., and Singer, B. 1998. The contours of positive human health. *Psychological Inquiry,* 9, 1–28.

Scanlan, T. K., Stein, G. L., and Ravizza, K. 1989. An in-depth study of former elite figure skaters: II. Sources of Enjoyment. *Journal of Sport and Exercise Psychology,* 11, 65–83.

Sheehan, G. 1983. *How to feel great 24 hours a day.* New York: Simon and Schuster.

Sheldon, K., and Kasser, T. 1998. Pursuing personal goals: Skills enable progress, but not all progress is beneficial. *Personality and Social Psychology Bulletin,* 22, 1270–79.

Shephard, R. 1999. Worksite fitness and exercise programs: A review of methodology and health impact. *American Journal of Health Promotion,* 10, 436–52.

Smuts, J. 1961. *Holism and evolution.* New York: Viking Press.

Bibliography

Sonstroem, R. 1997. The physical self-esteem: A mediator of exercise and self-esteem. In K. Fox, ed., *The physical self* (3–26). Champaign, Ill.: Human Kinetics.

Stedman, N. Apr. 13, 1999. A "flow" to fuel the reluctant athlete. *New York Times*, D7.

Stetson, B., Rahn, J., Dubbert, P., Wilner, B., and Mercury, M. 1997. Prospective evaluation of the effects of stress on exercise adherence in community-residing women. *Health Psychology, 16*, 515–20.

Strauss, R., and Miller, S. Feb. 19, 2001. Weighty problem. *People,* 65.

Strauss, R., et al. In press. Physical activity, self-efficacy, and self-esteem in healthy children. *Archives of Pediatric and Adolescent Medicine.*

Szabo, C., and Kimiecik, J. February 1997. *Flow and running*. Paper presented at the Midwest Sport and Exercise Psychology Conference, Ball State University, Muncie, Indiana.

Townsley, P. Summer 1996. Hold to the truth. *AWHP's Worksite Health,* 47.

Uchino, B., Cacioppo, J., and Kiecolt-Glaser, J. 1996. The relationship between social support and physiological processes: A review with emphasis on underlying mechanisms and implications for health. *Psychological Bulletin, 119,* 488–531.

U.S. Department of Health and Human Services. 1996. *Physical activity and health: A report of the Surgeon General.* Atlanta: U.S. Department of Health and Human Services, Centers for Disease Control and Prevention, National Center for Chronic Disease Prevention and Health Promotion.

U.S. House of Representatives, Committee on Ways and Means. 1998. *1998 Green book: Background material and data on programs within the jurisdiction of the Committee on Ways and Means.* Washington, D.C.: U.S. Government Printing Office.

Vallerand, R. J. 1997. Toward a hierarchical model of intrinsic and extrinsic motivation. In M. Zanna, ed., *Advances in experimental social psychology*, vol. 29 (271–360). New York: Academic Press.

Van Praag, H., Kempermann, G., and Gage, F. 1999. Running increases cell proliferation and neurogenesis in the adult mouse dentrate gyrus. *Nature Neuroscience, 2,* 266–70.

Bibliography

Walker, A. Apr. 5, 2001. *Baltimore Sun.*

Walsch, N. 1996. *Conversations with God.* New York: G. P. Putnam's Sons.

Wankel, L. 1985. Personal and situational factors affecting exercise involvement: The importance of enjoyment. *Research Quarterly for Exercise and Sport, 56,* 275–82.

White, R. 1959. Motivation reconsidered: The concept of competence. *Psychological Review, 66,* 297–333.

Wong, P. 1995. The process of adaptive reminiscence. In B. Haight and J. Webster, eds., *The art and science of reminiscing: Theory, research, methods, and applications* (23–35). Philadelphia: Taylor and Francis.

YMCA of the USA. *YPersonal Fitness Program: 12 Weeks to a Better You Program Manual.* Champaign, Ill.: Human Kinetics.

About the Author

Jay Kimiecik, Ph.D., is an associate professor at Miami University in Oxford, Ohio. He is a nationally known motivational speaker and the creator and host of *FitTalk*, a radio show on fitness and exercise. For the YMCA of the USA, he wrote the *YPersonal Fitness Program: 12 Weeks to a Better You*, an exercise behavior change program for physically inactive individuals that is used in more than 500 YMCAs in North America. He also wrote, directed, and produced the *YPersonal Fitness Program* video.

Kimiecik has published numerous studies in academic journals and conducted more than a hundred workshops and seminars. Along with Thelma Horn, he won the Research Writing Award, given by the Research Consortium of the American Alliance for Health, Physical Education, Recreation and Dance for his research published in *Research Quarterly for Exercise and Sport*. His practical writing has appeared in such magazines as *Runner's World, Psychology Today*, and the *IDEA Health and Fitness Source*.

An Invitation

I am always interested in hearing from people on issues relating to the intrinsic exerciser, motivation, self-discovery, and self-expression. I invite you to send your stories, questions, or comments to me via e-mail, phone, or fax.

Jay Kimiecik
PHS Department
Miami University
Oxford, OH 45056

513-529-2706 (w)
513-529-5006 (fax)
kimiecjc@muohio.edu